CW01481117

Preparing for Death
The Science of Dying

By C.W. Adams

Preparing for Death: The Science of Dying
Copyright © 2010 C.W. Adams
SCIENCE OF TRUTH PUBLISHING
Wilmington, Delaware
http://www.science-of-truth.com
All rights reserved.
Printed in USA
Front and back cover artwork by © Rolffimages

The information provided in this book is for educational and scientific research purposes only. The information is not medical or legal advice and is not a substitute for medical care or legal advice. A medical practitioner or other expert should be consulted prior to any significant change in diet, exercise or any other lifestyle change. There shall be neither liability nor responsibility should the information provided in this book be used in any manner other than for the purposes of education and scientific research.

Publishers Cataloging in Publication Data
Adams, Casey
Preparing for Death: The Science of Dying
First Edition
1. Science. 2. Philosophy
    Bibliography and References; Index

Library of Congress Control Number: 2010910560

ISBN 978-1-936251-09-4

For my Teachers,
who have taught me how to never die.

Table of Contents

Introduction

Every body dies. Each and every physical body comes to a point where it is no longer operable.

Yet most of us avoid the topic of death as though death could be avoided. As though death affects only some of us. As though some of us will somehow be able to dodge death, and only the unfortunate ones die.

When one of our relatives dies, we are shocked. It is as though it was never supposed to happen. Why did they have to be taken? As if the person who died should have never died.

As if none of us are supposed to die.

This book is about the reality of death. It is also a scientific foray into our real identities: Who are we, and what dies?

When one of our family members dies, we often will say, *"they are in a better place."* As their body lies before us in a casket, devoid of life, we pledge to our family that they are *"out there"* somewhere. Why are we clinging onto their life? Why must we be insistent that they are gone even though their body lies in front of us? And where is *"out there?"*

These are some of the many incongruities we find in our culture pertaining to death and identity. There are many, many other incongruities.

These are questions that take us into the realm of not only identity, but purpose. These questions, quite simply, are the essential questions of life. These are questions for which the answer cannot be vague or blurry. The answers must be clear. They must be scientific. They must be logical.

Here we will resolve these questions logically and scientifically. Here we will solve the riddle of death and just *who* is dying. We will also resolve the *whys* of death:

Why me? Why my wife or my husband? Why do we die and why are we born?

And most importantly, we will resolve the question of where we go: We will clarify, scientifically, what really is *"out there."*

1

Chapter One

Who Dies?

Death is defined by the Merriam-Webster dictionary as *"a permanent cessation of all vital functions: the end of life."* Therefore, to understand death, we need to understand when the life of the body ends. We also need to determine what life is.

What is Death?

In a medical sense, death has been a bit tricky. The conventional determination of death for many centuries was the stoppage of the heartbeat and the cessation of breath. In other words, once the heart stopped, and breathing stopped, the body was officially dead. And the time of death was recorded as the moment the breath and pulse stopped.

With the advent of new lifesaving techniques has come the ability to revive a person who stopped breathing. With CPR we can now manually restart the heart. CPR means cardiopulmonary resuscitation: Cardio refers to the heart and blood vessels, and pulmonary refers to breathing. So CPR means to bring the body that has stopped breathing or pumping blood back to life. The technique itself is basic: Begin breathing into the body's lungs at intervals to keep oxygen in the body—called rescue breathing—and periodically compress the chest to keep blood circulating. A Red Cross first aid course is recommended for further detail.

CPR is intended to circulate oxygen and blood to organs and tissues around the body until further medical treatment is available. This is because the body cannot typically be revived if the cells around the body, especially the brain, are not bathed in a constant flow of nutrients and oxygen. Once cells are cut off from nutrients, necrosis begins to take hold. Necrosis is the dying of the cells.

While some cells around the body can die without the whole body dying, the cells of the brain—especially those among the brain stem—are sensitive to necrosis. Once these neuron cells die, the whole body shuts down abruptly, followed by death.

In other words, the application of CPR and urgent care gradually led physicians and other professionals to the understanding that death does not necessarily take place when the breathing and heart stops. Since the heart and lungs can be restarted, death was found to be somehow aloof from these functions. As long as brain cells were not starved for oxygen and nutrients for too long the body could be revived—even if the heart and breath had stopped.

This led to the notion of *brain death*. Once the brain stops functioning, the person is now considered dead.

Following this realization, legal and medical institutions in the U.S. began to carefully define the moment of death to expel any confusion. They defined the moment a physician (and the law) could legally consider a person dead. State legislation in the United States began to define death with special statutes.

The first of these came in 1970 in the state of Kansas. Other states passed laws with sometimes differing criteria. In the 1970s, legal and health professional groups—notably the American Bar Association and the American Medical Association—attempted to create standards for death among their members. These led to several new state laws around the county, as the states began to adopt one standard. Some overrode, but others incorporated the older "common law" definition of death, which defined death as *"an absence of spontaneous respiratory and cardiac functions."* This led to many legal conflicts due to the advancement of resuscitation technologies. The new standards incorporated death as a loss of brain function: brain death became the new standard of defining death.

Eventually, the National Conference of Commissioners on Uniform State Laws created the *Uniform Determination of Death Act*. This 1981 act has now been adopted by most of the states, and has been approved by both the American Medical Association and the American Bar Association. The first and central statute of the act determines death as:

> *"An individual who has sustained either (1) irreversible cessation of circulatory and respiratory functions, or (2) irreversible cessation of all functions of the entire*

brain, including the brain stem, is dead. A determination of death must be made in accordance with accepted medical standards."

What is Life?

This is the big question. We know the body dies. We can easily observe that the body no longer functions. Regardless of which outward signs and symptoms we use, there is a dramatic change in the body at the time of death. The body ceases function. The body ceases the display of life and the outward demonstration of personality.

Where did this personality go then? Did it disappear into thin air? Did it evaporate with the final breath? Did this personality die with the death of the body?

Before we can fully understand death, we must understand life. What is a live person, and what is the difference between life and death? What is the difference between a dead body and a live body, and how is the personality we know and hold dear connected with life?

This means we must delve into the source of the energy and life of the body. Where is the generator of the body? Who or what is running the body? This certainly relates to the concept of *identity:* Are we each simply a temporary physical body? Are we simply cellular machines that decompose after a few decades?

If we ask someone who they are, they will most likely describe their body's physical features. Or perhaps their body's country of origin. They might say "I am American;" "I am black;" or "I am five feet tall, weigh 125 lbs, and female with brown eyes." The logical question here is: Am I this physical body? If so, what happens if the body gains 100 lbs of weight or becomes disfigured? Does my identity change?

Most of us assume that our identity runs deeper than our physical body. A person with a black body wants equality with a person with a white body because that person considers that beneath the skin, we are all of the same substance. Similarly, an obese person wants to be treated equally with someone of a more slender stature. Why would we request equality unless we are assuming we have deeper identities?

As science has debated this topic, there have been two general views (Popper and Eccles 1983): The first assumes a machine-like information-processing generating system with various modules of activity, all competing for control. This "chaos-machine" theoretically builds upon a system of learning and evolution without any central person or actor.

The other, more prevalent view historically, portrays the body as driven by an inner self or life force, central and governing to the body's existence. Among proponents of this inner self model, there is also some debate regarding the characteristics of the inner self. Some suggest it is a small part of the living organism. They refer to the "soul" as a type of "moral organ." Others refer to the soul as part of some kind of trinity: *"body, mind and spirit."* Still others consider the inner self as the central component of life. Debate on this topic continues, but empirical research data clarifies the conclusion.

The Living Force

Discerning the difference between a living body and a dead body was a topic of deep debate by the Greek philosophers. The existence of a living force separate from the body was promoted by many, including Plato, Aristotle, Ptolemy, Socrates, Hippocrates, Pythagoras, Origen and many others. Hippocrates professed that the life within the body was due to a "vital spirit" within, which acted through four different humors, for example.

When one of Socrates' students asked him how he wanted to be buried, Socrates gave them a clear reply: They could do whatever they wanted with the body, because he would be long gone by then.

By any physical observation made during the death of the body, the living force suddenly leaves. When we see a living body full of life, movement, energy, personality, and purpose, we understand these symptoms of life are residing within the body. When death arrives, suddenly those symptoms of life leave: There is no movement, no energy, and no personality remaining within the dead body. The body becomes lifeless. There is no growth, no will, no personality and no purposeful activity.

For thousands of years, doctors and scientists have autopsied, dissected and otherwise examined millions of dead bodies. No one—not even modern researchers with highly technical instruments—has been able to find any chemical or physical element missing from a dead body that was previously present when the body was alive. The dead body has every physical and material component the living body had. All of the cells are still there. The entire DNA is still there. All the nerves, the organs, the brain and central nervous system—every physical molecule and cell—are still resident in the cadaver.

The one and only claim of a difference, reported in 1907 by Massachusetts physician Dr. Duncan MacDougal, proposed a 21-gram weight difference between a dead and live body. He could not identify the substance of the difference, however. Dr. MacDougal's results were also inconsistent, and were never corroborated.

MacDougal's experiment consisted of monitoring six patients as they died upon a table rigged with a beam scale. Of the six, two were eliminated because of technical issues. Three subjects died of tuberculosis. Two of these were losing weight before and after death by *"evaporation and respiratory moisture."* One subject died from *"consumption"* and seemingly lost ¾ of an ounce in weight as he was dying—later converted to 21.3 grams. Dr. MacDougall admitted that it was difficult in some cases to know at what point the patient had died (MacDougall 1907).

A fellow doctor in Massachusetts, Dr. A. Clarke, immediately debated Dr. MacDougal's hypothesis. Dr. Clarke argued that the typical sudden rise in body temperature before and subsequent cooling without circulation upon death could account for slight weight changes due to evaporation. Especially noting some of the patients had lethal tuberculosis.

While Dr. MacDougal assumed the moment of death occured when the patient convulsed a bit and then lay still without breathing, modern research tells us that brain death must also occur—something Dr. MacDougal was not monitoring for.

Until his own death in 1920, Dr. MacDougall tried to repeat the results and could not confirm his findings. In one test, he cruelly killed fifteen dogs while weighing them and found no weight loss. No other study has substantiated such a theory of weight loss upon death. The 21-gram concept is now relegated to urban legend standards.

With the exception of these weak findings, many centuries of cadaver research and autopsy have carefully examined organs, bones, nerves, brain, blood, neurochemistry and other vital body parts. None has found any structural or biochemical difference between a live and dead body. The dead body is simply missing an immeasurable element of life that once animated the body: An invisible force that gives the body personality, energy, motivation, and the will to survive.

The life force of the body has never been seen under a microscope or by any other instrument. Furthermore, since this living force separates from the body at death—leaving the physical body with no life—it is obvious that this life force is not part of the body. Since the personality is also gone when this life is gone from the body, it would also be logical that our personality is part of this life force, and not part of the physical body. The physical body—including all the DNA and neurons—remains intact. Just as the driver is not the car: The driver can step out of the car at any time. Therefore, the driver has an identity separate from the car.

Which Body Part is Alive?

Following an amputation due to an infection or other injury, no one would claim the amputee is any less of a person. This is because the same personality is there despite a massive structural change in the body. This logic can be extended to even severe cases such as the loss of both arms and legs or other major parts of the anatomy. An explosion or other traumatic accident might leave ones torso intact while amputating both the body's arms and legs. Regardless of losing these appendages, the person is still perceived as a whole person—the same person as before—even though their body cannot function the way it did before. The person who operates the body still contains the same conscious being with the same personality. This is why paraplegic and quadriplegic rights are protected by law; and why Dr. Steven Hawking, a quadriplegic, is considered one of the today's foremost theoretical physicists despite his physical handicaps. He is regarded as no less of a person than the rest of us. Physically disabled people are given equal rights because society considers these persons equal in all respects, despite deficiencies in their physical bodies.

The physical organs illustrate the same logic. It is now commonplace in medicine to surgically remove and replace organs such as kidneys, livers, hearts, hips and other parts in order to preserve the healthy functioning of the body. Some parts—like hearts and hip sockets—are now replaced with artificial versions. Modern medicine has illustrated through many years of organ transplants that a person's identity does not travel with the organ. Otherwise, we might have—as a few comedic theatrical performances have suggested—people whose personalities reflect their organ donors. Imagine what would happen if someone receiving a heart transplant assumed part of the personality of the dead donor. We'd truly have a mess on our hands.

This situation is analogous to an auto accident: A car is involved in an accident and brought to an auto mechanic. The mechanic determines that the car needs a new set of tires, a new set of bumpers put on, and the engine rebuilt before the car can be put back on the road. The driver waits for the repairs to be completed, and then gets back in the car and drives it away. The new car parts do not affect the driver.

Matter versus Life

The difference between the physical body and the living personality requires a clear differentiation between matter and life. This investigation has been captured by science under the term *autopoiesis*. Autopoiesis is the study of the characterization of a complete living system as it compares to either a part of another living system or non-living matter.

To investigate this we could first analyze the difference between a living organism and a piece of matter without the component of life. An easy comparison would be between single-celled bacteria and a dead cell separated from a living body. A single-cell bacterium is a complete living organism. Studies have shown bacteria indeed respond to stimuli, avoid death, and avert pain. As we know from medicine, bacteria will intelligently mutate and adapt to antibiotics. Antibiotic-resistant superbugs are bacteria that have intelligently defended themselves. Living bacteria also conduct all of the activities required for independent survival: consumption, digestion, reproduction, self-propulsion, sense perception and emotional response, the intention to survive, and self-organization. Clive Backster's (2003) EEG work with bacteria proved that bacteria could sense danger through a subtle means of communication. This is also called quorum sensing. In quorum sensing, bacteria communicate amongst each other to come to consensus about the safety or risk about a particular environment.

Non-living objects display none of these characteristics. A machine may digest and respond to stimuli, but it will not have sense perception and emotional response. A machine relies upon a living person to program its tasking and response. Once a cell has been disconnected from a living organism, the cell ceases independent function.

A single cell can be put into a Petri dish and kept alive, however. This *in vitro* survival makes the cell now dependent upon the environment of the lab equipment, driven by living lab operators. The cell has thus become a surrogate of the lab, just as it was formerly a surrogate of the living body. It displays no independent sense perception, the desire to survive or independent emotional response. While the cell is part of the living body, it maintains the body's *self-concept*. Once detached, it displays metabolic continuation, but no separate self-existence.

Over many years of cruel laboratory research, test results have demonstrated that all animals and plants also have this self-concept awareness, which prevails through their responses to various environmental challenges. The functions of their mechanical physiology have also confirmed that this self-concept pervades through all living tissues, reflected by the display of episodic memory — remembering specifics about past events and past sensations. For this reason, we see animals learning quickly which activities result in pain and which activities result in pleasure. They immediately respond simply because every living being seeks pleasure (Dere *et al.* 2006).

Bitbol and Luisi (2004) sum up the distinction between living organisms and non-living matter as grounded within the principle of *cognition*. A definition of cognition as proposed by Bourgine and Stewart (2004) is, *"A system is cognitive if and only if sensory inputs serve to trigger actions in a specific way, so as to satisfy a viability constraint."* Bourgine and Stewart also contend *"A system that is both autopoietic and cognitive is a living system."* Bitbol and Luisi clarify that *"the very lowest level of cognition is the condition for life,"* and *"the lowest level of cognition does not reduce to the lowest level of autopoiesis."*

When we consider the element of cognition, we bring into focus the nature of awareness. Cognition is the awareness of *self* and *non-self*. The awareness of self and non-self are required for a living organism to consider survival important. Without an awareness of self and non-self, there is no intention for fulfillment. Without intention and the awareness of self, there is no consciousness. Without consciousness, there is no life.

Recycled Matter

Throughout its physical lifetime, our body is continually changing, yet we continue to maintain our core identity and consciousness. Research has shown all living cells in the body have a finite lifespan, ranging from minutes to days to years. A few cells — such as certain bone marrow stem cells and brain cells — may exist through the duration of the body. There are only a handful of these cells compared to the estimated 200 trillion cells making up the body, however. By far the vast majority of cells in the body will participate in cell division. Following division, older cells time out. They are broken down by the immune system and discarded, leaving the newly divided cells in their place.

Using this process the body constantly sloughs off older cells from the body, replacing them with new ones. Different cells in different parts of the body have different lifespans. For example:

- ❖ Gastric cells are replaced about every five minutes;
- ❖ Stomach lining cells are replaced within a week;
- ❖ Skin cells are replaced within about 90 days;
- ❖ The entire liver is regenerated within two months;
- ❖ The bone cells will all be replaced within a year.

While nerve cells and stem cells can live longer — for years — the composition of every cell, including all nerve and stem cells, undergoes an even faster turnover. Every cell in the body is made up of ionic and molecular combinations. These molecular combinations make up a cell's DNA, RNA, cytoplasm, organelles, and membrane. These atomic and molecular sub-units are constantly being replaced. New molecular matter enters the body from the environment. Old molecular matter is expelled through waste and respiration. Processes of cell membrane diffusion, osmosis and ionic channel conveyance allow each living cell to undergo a constant recycling of atomic elements.

Active cells will replace molecules and ions quite rapidly. Brain cells will recycle all their atoms and molecules within three days. Ninety-eight percent of all the atoms and molecules in the body are replaced within a year, and most biologists agree all the atoms and molecules within the body are replaced by new ones within five years.

Understanding that our physical bodies change nearly every cell within days, weeks or years; and all our body's atoms and molecules are being replaced from the food we eat, the water we drink and the air we breathe, we can accurately make the following statement:

The body we are wearing today is not the same body we were wearing five years ago.

We are now wearing a completely recycled body. In effect, we have each *changed bodies*. Every rhythmic element of matter — every vibrating atom — is different.

This might well be compared to a waterfall. The water within a waterfall is always changing. From moment to moment, the waterfall will be made up of different water. Therefore, the waterfall we see today is not the same waterfall we saw yesterday.

Since each of us is the same person from moment to moment and year to year within an ever-changing body, logically we each have an identity separate from this temporary vehicle. We cannot be the body, since the body has been replaced while we are still here. Should we look at our photograph taken five years ago, we will be looking at *a completely different body* from the one we are wearing today. The very eyes looking at the eyes in the picture are different.

Brain Recognition

One might propose that since we have yet to transplant someone's brain maybe we are the brain. Most of us have heard of the famous neurosurgical experiments first documented by Dr. Wilder Penfield, where he stimulated the temporal cortex and stimulated particular memories during brain surgery. These results and their confirmations left scientists with an impression that life must reside in the brain since emotional memories were stimulated with the electrode testing.

This assumption is disputed by other brain research over the past fifty years on both humans and animals, however. The assumption that the emotional self is contained in the brain has been conflicted by the many cases of emotions and memory following the removal of brain parts and even a majority of the brain. Mishkin (1978) documented that the removal of either the amygdala or the hippocampus did not severely impair memory. Mumby *et al.* (1992) determined that memory was only mildly affected in rats with hippocampus and amygdala lesions. According to a substantial review done by Vargha-Khadem and Polkey (1992), numerous hemidecortication surgeries—the removal of half the brain—had been conducted for a number of disorders. In a majority of these cases, cognition and brain function continued uninterrupted. A few cases even documented an improvement in cognition. Additionally, in numerous cases of intractable seizures, where substantial parts of brain have been damaged, substantial cognitive recovery resulted in 80 to 90% of the cases.

These and numerous other studies illustrate this effect— called *neuroplasticity*. In other words, the inner self is not reduced by brain damage or removal. The same person remains after brain parts are removed. The same personality remains. Many retain all their memories. The majority of brain-damaged stroke patients go about living normal lives afterward as well. Even in cases where memory, cognitive and/or motor skills are affected by cerebrovascular stroke, the person within is still present. Though handicapped, the person remains unaffected by the brain damage.

Memory, sensory perception and the emotional self-concept are not brain-dependent. Many organisms have memory and sensory perception without having a brain. Bacteria, for example, do not have brains, yet they can memorize a wide variety of skills and events, including what damaged or helped them in the past. Other organisms such as plants, nematodes and others maintain memory and recall without having brains or even central nervous systems.

MRI and CT brain scans on patients following brain injuries or strokes have shown that particular functions will often move from one part of the brain to another after the functioning area was damaged. We must therefore ask: Who or what is it that moves these physical functions from one part of the brain to another? Is the damaged brain area making this decision? That would not make sense. Some other guiding function must be orchestrating this move of the function. What or who is guiding this process?

The retention of memory, emotion, and the moving of brain function from one part of the brain to another is more evidence of a deeper mechanism; an *operator* or *driver* within the body who is *utilizing* the brain—rather than *being* the brain. The driver is the continuing element. Physical structures continually undergo change, while the driver remains, adapting to those changes.

The Elderly Contradiction

Consider how most of us perceive the aging of our body with respect to our identity. Most of us try to deny the age of our body in one respect or another. Teenagers want to be older and more mature, while older adults want to be younger and more youthful. Most adults refuse to accept getting old. As any birthday party will illustrate, adults are surprised at the body's age as it gets older. We try to disconnect ourselves from the physical age of our body somehow. This denial is often joked about, but to most of us—as we are faced with an ever-wrinkling body—it is no laughing matter. We are often embarrassed by our body's age as we get older. For this reason, many older adults do not want to state their age. They are embarrassed by it. They want to distance themselves from it. Furthermore, many of us dress the body with make-up, hair dyes and/or trendy clothes in an attempt to hide the body's age.

For this same reason, many in our society undergo extreme forms of surgery in order to achieve a younger looking body. In these cases, the self is in conflict with the images left by the body. Plastic surgery, hair-removal, hair transplantation, breast enhancement, and various other medical interventions are all extraordinary attempts to reconcile our identity with the temporary physical body.

In recent years, this struggle for self-identification has become more desperate for some, with people undergoing drastic surgery in an attempt to change their body's gender. Grotesque procedures such as sex organ replacement, combined with hormone injections, are sadly becoming commonplace in medical centers. Gender change is another stark example of how the self feels incompatible with the physical body.

Gender issues are controversial today. Women and men demand equal treatment regardless of physical or mental propensities. Homosexuals strive to erase prejudice in a predominantly heterosexual society. The struggles relating to identity and equality with regard to gender over the last few decades has led to childhood *gender confusion*. One recent report estimated as many as three million children in the U.S. suffer from gender confusion. In an attempt to accommodate this confusion and postpone a "decision," many of these children are prescribed hormone blockers to prevent normal puberty development. The concept is that hormone blocking will allow them to make a decision after they turn eighteen as to which gender they want to be—now that they have the option to undergo "corrective" surgery for a sex change.

Same-sex attraction and gender confusion is simply a symptom of incorrectly identifying the body with the self. Homosexuals illustrate this when they feel the only way to alleviate their inner struggle and confusion about their real identity is to 'come out,' and declare their homosexuality to others. This perceived self-identification problem has nothing to do with ones actual identity however. 'Coming out' does not alleviate the core issue causing the confusion. Their search to reconcile the body with the inner self continues after their 'coming out.'

Emotional Chemistry?

Over recent years, various researchers have proposed from one basis or another that our identities are chemical. They have proposed that emotions and personality are seated within the chemicals (such as hormones and neurotransmitters) that flow through the bloodstream, basal cell network and the synapses of our nervous systems. Could our identities simply be a mixture of complex chemicals? A logical review of the scientific evidence would indicate otherwise.

Emotional responses to environmental stimuli will initiate any number of biochemical cascade pathways to occur within the body. A cascade occurs when one chemical release stimulates the release of another biochemical, and that biochemical in turn stimulates the release of another. The biochemicals in the cascade might stimulate a particular cell, tissue or organ function. With each cascade, there are initiating stimuli and subsequent responses from various tissues and nerves.

Because neurologists and other researchers have seen these biochemicals involved with emotional response, some have proposed that these biochemicals contain the emotion. They propose that chemicals such as endorphins, dopamine, serotonin, epinephrine, or acetylcholine each contain the particular emotions they reflect, and are thus the sources of the emotion. They propose that these signaling biochemicals connect with receptors positioned at the surface of the cell; and the response by the cell is the emotion being released from the chemical. An example some have used is the famed *opiate receptor,* linked with the cell's reception of morphine or endorphins, and the sensation of euphoria. The idea is that the feeling of euphoria is produced when the ligands like endorphin connect with the receptor.

One problem with this speculation is that no two organisms respond identically to the same chemical. With opiates for example, some may hallucinate while others may only respond casually. On the other hand, some may have nightmarish experiences. If these structurally identical neurochemicals *contained* the emotion, why would each person respond differently to the same chemical and dose?

Another major problem with this thesis is the observer: *Who* is observing that the body is feeling euphoria? *Who* observes the hallucinations created by certain chemicals? *Who* observes the positive or negative sensations of the body? The fact is, without an observer, there is no way to be able to view feelings. A physical body that is experiencing a physical emotional response with no observer could not observe and review the experience. Therefore, there could be no discretion regarding the event. There could be no judgment available as to whether the experience was positive or negative. There could be no available decision on whether the experience should be repeated or curtailed. There could be no analysis or learning experience from our activities. These require an observer of the experience.

The perception of pain may offer some clarity. In 2005, Dr. Ronald Melzack, co-author of the now-standard 1965 *gate control theory* of pain transmission, updated his theory of pain from a simple gateway effect to one of a multidimensional experience of *neurosignatures.* His new theory—which he calls the *body-self neuromatrix*—explains that the consensus of clinical research over thon acute pain, behavior and chronic pain indicates an independent perceptual state of self; observing and exchanging feedback and response with the locations of injury. Because doctors and researchers have found a good portion of the pain response is unrelated to specific injury but rather a modification of sensory experience, this *neuromatrix* indicates that pain requires an interaction between the nervous system and what Melzack calls the *"self."*

In other words, pain requires two components: 1) The sensory transmission of pain and 2) the observer or experiencer of that pain. Once that pain is experienced, there may also be a feedback response from the experiencer. This feedback may either be: 1) take action to remove the cause of the pain; or 2) if there is no apparent cause then become extra-sensitive to the pain until the cause is determined (Baranauskas and Nistri 1998). This increased sensory elevation leads to what is called *nociceptic pain* – pain not appearing to have a direct physical cause. Some might also refer to this type of pain as being *psychosomatic,* although psychosomatic pain is often considered not real. Noiceptive pain is considered real, but its cause is not obviously physically apparent.

Regardless of the name, this type of pain is very difficult to understand and manage. This is especially true for doctors and patients who deal with chronic pain that appears unrelated to trauma or inflammation. Because the self naturally seeks pleasure, we would propose that the current cause of that pain is always real, from either a gross physical level or a more subtle level. Regardless of the level, the self experiencing the pain would certainly be considered separate from the pain, along with any biochemical messengers assisting in its transmission. After all, how could the self "escape" pain unless it was separate from the cause of the pain? Because they increase the separation of the self from the pain source, pain medications are a multi-billion dollar business.

Since the biochemical transmission effectors such as *substance P* among neurons are present during pain responses, it is logical that these chemicals have a *role* in the physical responses to emotions or memories. However, the proposal made by scientists such as Candace Pert, Ph.D. that emotions exist *within* the chemicals is not supported by logic or observation.

Researchers have observed an increase in biochemicals like dopamine, serotonin, and various endorphins in the bloodstream during feelings of love or compassion. The question being raised is whether the emotions stimulated the biochemicals or the biochemicals stimulated the emotions. The implications of proposing the limited view that the emotion was created by the biochemicals are many. This would be equivalent to saying love comes from biochemicals. It would open the door to a murder suspect pleading that his body's chemical balance was responsible for his committing the fatal crime.

Dopamine, serotonin and endorphins are circulating at heightened levels following activities such as laughing eating, sex and post-traumatic stress. These biochemicals are also circulating at other times, during other emotions, albeit at different levels. What comes first, the biochemical or the emotion? Does the emotion drive the biochemical levels or do the biochemicals drive the emotional response? To break this down properly, we must separate the physiological response to an optional response relating to optional behavior and decision-making. Yes, a biochemical reaction or ligand-receptor response can stimulate a physiological response. But can it dictate behavior? Could a hormone or neurotransmitter ligand-receptor response force us to shoplift? In that case, we should be able to find that certain biochemicals were "shoplifting" chemicals. We'd be able to just reduce their levels and forget about putting shoplifters in jail. We'd also have to look at blood donors' criminal records before accepting their blood.

The reason we put shoplifters in jail is to teach them that shoplifting is morally wrong. This is decision for an observer — an inner self — who can observe the body's activities. Each of us can observe our activities and steer them with decision-making. We may not always be able to steer our physiological responses, which also produce certain moods within the brain and nerves. But we can observe those moods and decide whether we are going to let them control our activities. While more shoplifters are likely to have bad moods, we aren't forced to shoplift by a bad mood.

If biochemicals create emotion, they would be present only in and prior to particular emotions. Instead, they are present during a variety of emotions. Again physiological changes can be brought about by biochemicals. But emotions stem from life: There is no emotion left in a dead body.

Furthermore, if chemicals could contain emotions, these emotional characteristics should exist in the chemicals both inside and outside of the particular body of the person experiencing the emotion. Illustrating this, health workers regularly remove biochemicals (in the form of body fluids such as blood, plasma and marrow) from one subject and transfer them (or their components) to other subjects. In none of these cases are emotions transferred from one person to another. Supposed "emotional biochemicals" do not retain or display the emotions of their donor once they are transferred to a new host. Certainly, if we found that blood transfusions resulted in changes in personality or emotions, blood transfusions would not be very popular.

Thus, the basis for a biochemical self fails thousands of times a day around the world in hospitals that transfuse blood.

This is not to mean that injected biochemicals cannot stimulate a physical response within a new host, which may or may not facilitate particular emotions to be expressed. The organism receiving epinephrine or another neurochemical may experience a physical response consistent with the *vanilla* biochemical response related to that particular molecular structure. Injected adrenaline may produce a physical reaction of increased heart rate, for example. However, adrenaline drawn from one person during a fearful response will not induce a recall of the donor's fears. The recipient's physical response after the injection will neither reflect the appropriate response required for the donor's particular fears.

Once the inner self responds to a particular sensory input—often signaled through biochemical reception—the unique emotional response of the self stimulates particular biochemicals to translate and express the emotion. In other words, these biochemicals help *translate* the emotional self's response.

Just as current travels within an electrical wire, neurotransmitters help transmit sensory feedback messages to the inner self. They also help transmit emotional responses from the inner self. The self is the observer of sensory input, and stimulates feedback responses utilizing some of the same biochemical transmission pathways.

We must therefore conclude that there is someone inside who is either—directly or indirectly—receiving and responding to the body's neural transmissions. Any response that proceeds with direction and decision-making must come from a conscious source. Otherwise we would simply be machines.

Fuel may ignite a spark in the cylinder of an automobile engine causing combustion, which will push the rods into motion, exerting force on the axel cranks. Fuel is not the original stimulant, however. Nor does fuel contain the ability to guide and steer the car. Rather, there is a driver within the car who consciously turns the key and drives the car to a particular destination using the steering wheel, accelerator, and brakes. The driver optionally stimulates the flow of fuel through the injection system. The driver can also stop the flow of fuel by turning off the car.

When the driver of the body leaves at the time of death, there are no emotions exhibited in the dead body. Yet all the hormones, neurotransmitters, genes and cells—all the biochemical ligands and receptors—are still contained within the recently dead body. The body supports no memory or emotional response because there is no longer a conscious driver present. The conscious driver who drove the feedback and response neurochemistry has left.

Emotions elicited from a response to an observation or other sensual stimuli would logically come from someone separate from those stimuli. Because emotion is integral with interpreting stimuli, an observer would be necessary for that interpretation.

Without an observer, there could be no decision-making: There would be no optional behavior.

This does not mean that all physiological responses require conscious interpretation and decision from the self. For example, should we touch the burner of a stove there is programming in place within the neural network to instantly react by pulling the hand away. This will often happen before the self has a chance to make a decision. However, this programming does not mean the self cannot engage in the decision to resist that reaction of pulling away. A firewalker may intentionally walk on the coals despite his sympathetic system's programmed response to jump away onto the cool sand. These observations lead us to understand that the self can be involved in almost any sensory reception should there be determination and intention.

Most other stimuli requires the emotional self to respond. Otherwise, no action would occur. This is where intention comes in. Upon hearing the alarm in the morning, the self could choose to do nothing—lying in bed for the rest of the day. The self could also intend to accomplish something that day, and rise to begin the day's activities. Ultimately, the self creates the intention and impetus for those activities.

While biochemicals participate in the process of conscious response and feedback, they are actually conductors for electromagnetic wave transmissions. Once sensual stimuli are pulsed to the neural network after ligand reception, neurons produce specific information waves. As we will discuss later in more depth, at any particular point in time, there are billions of brainwaves of various frequencies moving through the brain. As the different waves collide—or interfere—they create different types of interference patterns. The neurological research headed up by Dr. Robert Knight at the University of California at Berkeley and UC at San Francisco illustrated that the interaction of these interference patterns together formulate a type of informational transmission and mapping system.

This mapping system forms a type of observational screen from which the self can view incoming waveform information. Using this mapping system, the self can view the sensory information coming in from sense organs, and combine these with the feedback from the body, creating a total perception of ones environment and situation.

As the self views these waveform interference pattern images, we can respond with intention. Intention from the self is typically translated through the prefrontal cortex and medial cortex to create brainwave patterns that express the self's response. These response brainwave patterns are translated through the hypothalamus and pituitary gland to produce master hormones such as growth hormone, adrenocorticortropic hormone, follicle-stimulating hormone, oxytocin, luteinizing hormone, and others, stimulating the cascade of biochemicals that translate the response into action. The brainwave transmissions also stimulate a particular nervous system response which activate particular muscles, organs and other tissues. The end result is a physical action combined with certain biochemicals that stimulate a physical response.

We can illustrate this process more practically. Let's say that we heard from a friend that a relative was hurt. The transmission brought through our body's ears will cause an emotional reaction from us as soon as we hear it. The emotion was experienced following the aural reception of the announcement. Upon interpreting the aural reception, our inner self—we—react emotionally. The particular response would depend upon our personal connection with the relative. It is not automatic. If they were a vicious, hurtful relative, we may react far differently than if they we had established a close personal relationship with them.

Assuming a close personal relationship, our inner self may then initiate a physical response, producing tears and a rush to the hospital to be with them. These physical activities were stimulated by the emotional response of our inner self. The emotional response and subsequent activities were optional responses made by a conscious individual. It would be nonsensical to say that this was a biochemical response. Why would a group of unconscious biochemicals have a problem with another group of remotely located biochemicals?

The Observer

Consider biofeedback. Sensors are attached to various parts of the body to monitor physical responses like heart rate, breathing, brainwaves, skin response, muscle activity, and so on. These sensors are connected to a computer, which displays the various response levels onto a monitor for the subject to see. The heart rate amplitude and frequency readings will be displayed on the monitor in waves, bars, and/or numbers. With a little practice, most people—once they see their heart rate with graphics clearly on the monitor—can consciously lower their heart rate with intention. Biofeedback has thus been used successfully to teach people to alter physical functions such as muscle tension, hunger, physical stress, and other autonomic functions. Biofeedback training also gives the subject the ability to directly control a variety of physical issues, including stomach cramps, muscle spasms, headaches, and others—many known to be part of a biochemical cascade.

The reason why the biofeedback subject can learn to control certain autonomic functions is that the self ultimately exists outside of these bodily functions. The self is the key participant who influences physical functions. Once the person intends to make a change, the mind will facilitate the stimulation of the biochemicals by the appropriate glands to produce a physiological response. This can take time, discipline and practice. Even without biofeedback, a person can initiate various autonomic responses. Most of us have experienced how a physiological fear response may be initiated by simply imagining a dangerous event or situation. This happens every day in the professional world, where executives stress over events that may never happen. Stress increases the heart rate and stimulates stress-biochemical release. Most of us have experienced being worried about an event that may never happen. The resulting increase in our heart rate indicates our body's autonomic response to an over-anxious self.

If the self can affect the body's biochemistry with anxiousness, the self is separate from the biochemistry. Furthermore, if the self can affect the body's biochemistry intentionally, there is no question of the self's ability to direct the body through intention. The range of control the self has over the body is limited by design. Still, there is no doubt that intention initiates the sequencing of instructional signaling through the body.

This neurochemical process would be analogous to a computer operator operating a computer. A computer will tabulate, calculate, and memorize data. It will display various graphics and perform various functions, based upon the input or direction of the operator. The software and hardware are designed in such a way to coordinate computer functions very quickly and automatically within particular limitations. Regardless of the programming, the operator is required. The computer operator must decide to turn on the computer and must decide to input into the machine certain intentional commands to initiate the computer's programming functions. In the same way, the physical body, with all of its functional chemistry and various physical responses, is ultimately being steered by the personality within: this is the self, the living being — the operator of the body.

It is difficult sometimes to separate the self inside the body from the various physical and biochemical operations of the body. This is because the feedback-response system bridges the self with the physical body. For example, breast-feeding is now being rediscovered. Researchers have discovered that breast-feeding not only gives the child better nourishment and a stronger immune system, but also stimulates brain development due to some of the biochemistry of breast milk. This notion is consistent with the role various nutrients or drugs have in altering moods and behavior.

Chemicals influence behavior because they not only stimulate physical tissue response, but they also give feedback to the self about what is going on in the body. For example, the feeling of thirst is a neurochemical signal to the self that the body needs water. The combination of hormonal, osmotic, ionic and nerve signaling all integrate to stimulate *osmoreceptors* located among brain tissue (such as the anteroventral third ventricle wall). Once stimulated, these receptors initiate waveform signaling through the hypothalamus, which converts into the more subtle wave-forms of the mind. Through the reciprocation of the mind, the self observes this feedback, and responds by initiating action to find some water.

A computer will also feed back to its operator in the same way. The computer is not only designed to perform operations based upon the input of the operator, but also its programming is designed to feed back to the operator the results of those operations, signaling a need for new responses from the operator.

This process is called a feedback loop. The body's feedback system is designed to respond to environmental and physical changes around the anatomy. The system is designed to signal to the self on how the body is functioning. This is one of the purposes for serotonin release in the body: To feed back the presence of balance within particular organs and tissue systems. A diet balanced in proteins, carbohydrates, and fats, along with physiological activities stimulate the conversion of tryptophan to serotonin. This conversion is also stimulated by such activities as relaxation, laughter, and exercise. These are all positive activities for the body's metabolism. This combined state of balance and activity results in a normal flow of serotonin, which feeds back through the brain's translation systems to the self the presence of physiological balance among certain parts of the body.

Pain, on the other hand, indicates quite the opposite: Some imbalance exists somewhere. Pain feeds back to the operator the need for an adjustment among certain functions or activities. This necessary adjustment could be to the diet, fluid intake, sitting posture, lack of exercise, or perhaps an infection of some sort. Chronic pain indicates an unresolved lack of balance in the body, requiring an appropriate response to fix the issue.

Just as an instrument panel on an automobile informs the driver of the running condition of car, we can monitor the condition of our body through these and other neurochemical feedback mechanisms. Just as the car driver slows down when the speedometer shows the car is over the speed limit, the self—directly through conscious control or indirectly through the autonomic system—can make the needed adjustment when the body's feedback systems indicate a problem.

Should we misidentify ourselves as the body, we might confuse positive feedback mechanisms as pleasure. This misconception leads us to attempt to manipulate our body's biofeedback mechanisms. Eating, for example, will stimulate neurochemicals such as serotonin, dopamine and leptin when there is a balance of nutrition and energy. Another example is how our taste buds feed back positive neural signals when we eat something sweet or fatty. These are both positive responses to the body achieving its basic fuels.

In an effort to gain pleasure from these positive responses, many of us continue to eat long after the body has enough for its fuel. An ongoing attempt to become fulfilled through eating can result in obesity, frustration, and depression. In the same way, the car driver does not get full when he fills the car's fuel tank. Thus, the answer to obesity is the realization of this conflict between the body's fulfillment and the fulfillment of the self.

> *"Happiness resides not in possessions and not in gold;*
> *the feeling of happiness dwells in the soul."*
> - Democritus ("The father of science," 4th
> century, B.C.)

Genetic Anomaly

A newer version of biochemical identity put forth by scientists over the last few decades is the notion that the self is the genetic information—or DNA—of the body.

The assumption that we are DNA is buried within the theory that genes accidentally evolved from chemicals. The gene evolution theory supposes that genes, and life itself, spontaneously arose from a random pool of chemicals. This theory requires a process called *spontaneous generation*. Unlikely as it seems, the spontaneous generation of life theory was debated by scientists for hundreds of years, as they observed life seemingly growing from barren flasks. Finally, Dr. Louis Pasteur refuted spontaneous generation by illustrating that this growth was due to the presence of tiny microorganisms invisible to the naked eye. For many decades this assumption has continued nonetheless. Many researchers have attempted to create life from 'primordial' chemicals — all without success.

To analyze the likelihood of even one typical protein molecule to have been randomly developed, we can reference Dr. Francis Crick's statements in his 1981 book *Life Itself: Its Origin and Nature.* Here Dr. Crick calculates that the chance of even one conservative protein molecule of two hundred amino acids coming into existence is one chance in 10^{260} — the number one with two hundred and sixty zeros behind it. He furthermore states that this would be analogous to a billion monkeys typing onto a billion typewriters and somehow typing one sonnet of Shakespeare.

The chance of a 1,000-nucleotide chain DNA molecule forming accidentally is more remote. Both Dr. Dawson and Dr. Crick agree with this. Lester Smith (1975) calculated the probability as about one in 10^{600}.

The probability of genetic mutations accidentally leading to a new species is even more remote. Dr. Lee Spetner (1998) calculates that a new species (one positive mutation step) would have a (negative) probability of 2.7×10^{-2739}, using Stebbins' (1966) estimation that five hundred intermediate mutations would be required to establish one positive mutation step.

This fantastic assumption that chemicals spontaneously (even a gradual development is still considered spontaneous without a determined cause) created genes and life assumes also that the chemicals combined somehow developed the *desire to survive.* In other words, these chemical combinations somehow developed the intention to improve their chances of survival. Have we ever observed chemicals desiring survival? Chemicals simply do not display this characteristic. No scientist has ever found the intent to survive outside of a living organism. No chemical desires survival unless part of a living organism — hence the name *biochemicals* (bio = life). Chemicals may react and form various substances, and certainly will change structure when heated or cooled. Having a desire to survive is another matter altogether.

The desire to survive is connected to the desire to improve survival factors and eliminate threats to survival. The need to improve survival requires that *someone* values survival over death. Otherwise, we would be talking about a group of unconscious chemicals somehow beginning to value their existence.

Chemicals that value their own existence means that the chemicals could somehow recognize a difference between *living* chemicals and *dead* chemicals. This in turn requires that chemicals have *awareness,* because the desire to survive requires an awareness of self-existence. It also requires a fear of death: Could a chemical become afraid to die?

In order to desire survival, a living organism must be aware that it is alive. A living organism must be able to differentiate itself from a dead batch of chemicals. If there is no distinction between life and death, why avoid death? Why desire life without a distinction between living and nonliving chemicals? Certainly it would be easier for a batch of chemicals to remain dead than to have to struggle for survival in the midst of all the environmental challenges to staying alive.

A small unicellular organism can be killed by so many environmental challenges: Freezing, direct sun exposure and any number of natural enemies. If there were no distinction between living or dead chemicals, the path of least resistance would be to remain dead chemicals. Why try to survive without a benefit for living? If there were no awareness and desire for survival in the face of all this resistance, there would be no incentive for genes to develop and evolve towards greater complexity — the basic tenet of the evolutionary theory and the 'survival of the fittest.'

Put more simply, if a living entity could not distinguish itself from a nonliving entity, there would be no urge to survive. Without the urge to survive, there would be no motivating factor to encourage adaptation or mutation. There would be no impetus to evolve because survival is not valuable without an awareness of life.

In his 1977 book *The Selfish Gene,* Dr. Robert Dawkins proposed that genes themselves somehow became not only selfish in their orientation, but also somehow acted upon their selfishness. Certainly, we can all agree that in order to become "selfish," there must be a "self." Without a self, how could something become *self*ish? How could there be an orientation towards one-*self* without there being a self?

We must also ask, logically, just *who* would be available to recognize life in a chemical-based existence? We are being asked to assume a batch of chemicals developed a state of consciousness, yet there is no individual present the chemicals to be conscious of being alive?

The incidental gene theory of life simply has no logical basis. Genes cannot desire survival. They cannot mutate, or make changes that promote survival without a conscious self present within the organism who values life. This living being must be aware that it is alive, and must therefore value survival. Once the self values survival, it has a logical basis for making genetic and physiological adjustments to better adapt to the environment. Because the self is fundamentally alive when it is inserted into a temporary physical body, it naturally strives to survive within that organism.

Admittedly, the total mapping of the genome and further mapping of the individual allele locations within codons — their haplotypes and collectively, their hapmaps — reveals a complexity of design beyond our current understanding.

Over the past three decades, tremendous research efforts have gone into creating statistical models to match the physical traits of humans and other organisms with particular gene sequences. As a result, thousands of species genomes have been tabulated and connected with physical characteristics.

In addition, different diseases have been connected to certain sequences. Although these efforts are laudable, science has unfortunately succumbed to a blurring of the relationship between these genetic traits and life itself. The erroneous assumption is that gene sequences — the particular arrangement of alleles or nucleotides at different positions of the DNA molecule — are the *cause* of those physical or behavioral traits. That somehow, those sequences together make up the identity of the individual.

While some might call this a chicken-and-egg problem, the solution is certainly clearer than this. This assumption that the self is the genetic hapmap would be equivalent to saying a telephone is the source of the voice we hear through its speaker. It is elementary: The voice on the line is coming from a remotely located person. We may not be able to see the person while we are speaking with them, but we know a person is out there because we exchange personal communication and perform a type of voiceprint analysis as we hear their voice. In addition, the voice on the other side responds to our statements with a clarity that can only come from a conscious speaker. Even computerized voice greetings are clearer if they are recorded by real people.

The sequencing of genetic haplotypes indicates its complex structure. This complex coding indicates programmed design. As with any programming, there must be an underlying motive for the program. It is not logical to assume that a complex, well-designed code with specific rules comes from a chaotic and accidental design process. Just as we can connect the lucid voice on the phone to a personal consciousness, we can tie the sequencing of genes to a living, intentional component, ultimately driving its design with intention.

If we were to extract a DNA molecule from our skin or body fluids, and place it onto the table or even in a test tube, we will find there is no display of life. Just as the body after death is lifeless, DNA or RNA molecules extracted from a living body become lifeless. It should also be clarified that RNA transcription and genetic mutation is impossible without a living being driving the process. We can certainly force a mutation upon an organism or its seed through the vehicle of a virus. Yet the mutation will only become duplicated through an organism if there is a living force present in that organism. In other words, we cannot insert a mutated gene into a dead body and see that mutation replicated through the dead body.

The proposal that personality is determined by genetic code is refuted by children who have inherited genes from parents.

Children are each born with distinct personalities, talents and character traits not necessarily portrayed in their parents or grandparents. While we are quick to notice similar physical traits among our children, each has their own character and personality. We can easily observe children behaving significantly different from their parents in similar situations. We can also witness the many conflicts that arise between children and parents. We have also observed that the extraordinary talents of child music geniuses or savants are not passed down genetically. In most musical savant cases, the parents have relatively little or no musical gift whatsoever.

If personality and behavior were genetically driven then genetically identical twins would live parallel lives and have identical personalities. They would make the same decisions, leading to identical histories.

This is not supported by the research. Twins live dramatically unique and individual lives from each other. Depending upon how much time they spend together, they will make distinctly different choices in life as well. In general, they display significantly unique and often diverse behavior. Hur and Rushton (2007) studied 514 pairs of two to nine year old South Korean monozygotic and dizygotic twins. Their results indicated that 55% of the children's pro-social behavior related to genetic factors and 45% was attributed to non-shared environmental behavior. It should also be noted that shared environmental factors could not be eliminated from the 55%, so this number could well be higher if shared environments were removed.

In another study from Quebec, Canada (Forget-Dubois *et al.* 2007), an analysis of 292 mothers demonstrated that maternal behavior only accounted for a 29% genetic influence at 18 months and 25% at 30 months. In a study of 200 African-American twins, including 97 identical pairs, genetics accounted for about 60% of the variance in smoking (Whitfield *et al.* 2007). In a study done at the Virginia Commonwealth University's Institute for Psychiatric and Behavioral Genetics (Maes *et al.* 2007), a large sampling revealed that individual behavior was only about 38-40% attributable to genetics, while shared environment was 18-23% attributable and unshared environmental influences were attributable in 39-42%. These studies are also confirmed by others, illustrating a large enough variance from 100% to indicate the presence of an individual personality within each twin.

Distinct identity despite genetic sameness is further evidenced by the fact that identical twins will have distinctly different fingerprints, irises and other physical traits, despite their identical genetics. Many twins also differ in handedness and specific talents. Researchers have found that twins will often have significantly different lifestyle choices later in life such as sexual preference, drug abuse, and alcoholism.

For example, say two people purchase the exact same make, model and year automobile at the same time. Comparing the two cars in the future will reveal the cars had vastly different engine lives and mileages. They each had different types of breakdowns, and different problems. This is because each car was driven differently. One was likely driven harder than the other was. One was likely better taken care of than the other was. They may have been the same make and model, but each had different owners with different driving habits.

Because twins have the same genetics—just as the cars shared the same make and model—the unique factors related to the eventual circumstances of their lives stem from the fact that each body contains a distinct driver.

Because geneticists are not aware of the inner self, they are now trying to resolve the inherent inconsistencies of the gene theory with the developing theories of epigenetics. In general, epigenetics is the acceptance of additional factors (called *marks* or *phenotypes*) that affect the switching on or switching off of genes. This is also called gene expression. It was hypothesized—and confirmed by research—that while the DNA may or may not change within a species, there are many physiological and anatomical changes that will take place within a lifetime or within immediate generations that will reflect environmental changes. These environmental changes are seen as turning on or off these phenotypes, enabling changes in the epigenome of the individual or family.

The concept of epigenetics was proposed by geneticist Conrad Waddington in the early 1940s to explain how environmental circumstances could effect genetic expression. In the 1980s, Dr. Lars Olov Bygren studied Northern Sweden populations that descended from families who were isolated and subjected to periodic famines. He found that children of famines had different genetic traits than those who did not live through famine. Those who lived through periodic feast and famine years died sooner and had more cardiovascular disease.

As researchers have discovered more genetic anomalies—such as the twins research mentioned earlier—the concept of epigenetics has received increasing attention.

The biochemical relationships between gene expressions have focused upon the action of DNA methylation or histone regulation. These biochemical messengers have been implicated in the process of switching alleles on or off. The assumption once again has been that the body's switching systems are purely mechanical and robotic. There is no intentional driver or observer present: Only a biochemical machine that somehow acts with desire and direction.

However, the very research by geneticists that theoretically supported epigenetics also exposed a major shortfall in the theory. In cruel mice experiments at McGill University's Douglas Hospital Research Center (Szyf *et al.* 2008), epigenetic phenotypes could be turned on and off within baby mice by the increased nurturing from the mother. In other words, baby mice receiving mama's nurturing would switch on genes differently than mice not receiving nurturing from mama mouse.

Quite simply, this indicates the presence of another influence upon the genetic switching of epigenetic phenotypes: That of an exchange between emotional personalities. Nurturing is, in its very essence, the expression of love between one living being and another. When a mother communicates love through nurturing, the baby receives that expression of love through those nurturing activities. As the expression is received, there is a resonation or hand-shaking between the two living beings. That resonation produces an effect upon genetic expression through the pathways of the brain, nervous system and the body's bio-chemicals, which bridge the self with the body and its genes.

The inner self is also connected to the body's genes through conscious decision-making. The research has quite resoundingly connected environmental changes with epigenetic changes. Yet many environmental changes are the direct result of the decisions of the inner self.

Let's say we decided that we wanted to live in a warm climate. Furthermore, we decided that a warm climate was more important to us than having a good job. So we packed up our belongings and moved to Hawaii. We settled down in Hawaii and lived there for the next twenty years. Over that time, our body will undergo many adjustments as it accommodates the warm, humid weather of Hawaii. Eventually, these environmental conditions will affect the switching on and off of certain genes, ultimately changing our genetic outcome. One might be a longer life. Epidemiological research has confirmed that Hawaii residents have the longest life expectancy among other states in the U.S.—at 80 years—while the average life expectancy of the rest of the country is 78.3 years. Without our conscious decision to give up our job and move to Hawaii, those physical (and epigenetic) results would never have occurred.

The bottom line is that epigenetics research illustrates that we are not the genes: We are the living being within, who can affect and change our genes with our conscious choices.

The Inner Self

Empirical and clinical evidence reveals the existence of a transcendental inner self operating the body. Why do we say "transcendental?" If the self were not transcendental to the physical plane we would be able to see it. We would be able to measure it with physical quantifications. As it is, we can only see it in the animation of the body. We can only see it through the emotions that are expressed through the body. We can only see it in the decision-making and objectives that push the body to act one way or another. It is, in fact, the inner self's transcendental nature that has caused modern science to completely ignore the existence of the self.

The inner self is the source of personality and life, which the body expresses through physical activity over its lifetime. There is energy, personality and movement in a living body prior to death. This is followed by a lack of movement, personality and energy after the death of the body. This means that the source of the energy and personality must leave the body at death.

Furthermore, contrary to the proposals of many, since each personality is unique and different from everyone else, each inner self must also be an independent, individual being. We are not, despite the seductiveness of such a statement, "all one."

Consistent with the ancient teachings of all major religions, the ancient philosophers, and the vast majority of western scientists prior to the emergence of the accidental chemical life theory, we can now scientifically and empirically document the existence of a unique individual being, transcendental to the gross physical plane.

Plato, Socrates and most of the ancient Greek philosophers referred to this inner self as the *soul*. The translation is thought to originate with Aristotle, who described the self with the Latin *telos*. Rather than a vague spirit-like organ, *telos* translates to a personality with purpose, will, and character. In this context, we would emphasize that each of us does not possess a soul: each of us *is a soul* – accessing the physical plane through a temporary physical body.

We conclude this discussion with a comment made by the fifteenth-century physician, Paracelsus:

> *"The power to see does not come from the eye, the power to hear does not come from the ear, nor the power to feel from the nerves; but it is the spirit of man that sees through the eye, hears with the ear, and feels by means of the nerves. Wisdom and reason and thought are not contained in the brain, but belong to the invisible spirit which feels through the heart and thinks by means of the brain."*

Chapter Two

The Death of the Mind

The mind is one of the most misunderstood aspects of the human condition. Is the self the mind? Is the mind the self? And if the mind is not the self, then what is it? And if the self is not the mind, then does the mind die when the body dies? These are critical questions. It is essential that we are clear about the nature and function of the mind. In order to be prepared for death, we must understand the role the mind plays in life and death.

Mind versus Self

There has been a great movement over the last century proposing that the mind is the person, and is therefore inseparable form the self. Furthermore, many of these proponents have conjectured that thoughts have the capacity to control the physical world. This was proposed a century ago by William Walker Atkinson in the book *Thought Vibration or the Law of Attraction in the Thought World* (1906). The proposals put forth by Atkinson in this and almost one hundred other books — some under a variety of pseudonyms — are similar. Atkinson's theory has formed the framework for a multitude of self-help books in the decades following and to the present day. Atkinson's theory attracted a number of followers, including influential writers such as Mary Baker Eddy of *Christian Science* fame and Wallace Wattles, author of *The Science of Getting Rich* (1910). The *governing mind* philosophy of the late Mr. Atkinson and Mr. Wattles has also influenced various other works, such as *Think and Grow Rich* (1937) by Napoleon Hill, *The Greatest Salesman in the World* (1968) by Og Mandino, and the wildly popular book and movie, *The Secret* (2006) by Rhonda Byrne.

These works have attracted the masses because of their promise of material successes such as wealth and admiration. These appeals to our more narcissistic natures appear to be grounded in the idea seemingly first proposed by Atkinson: The self is the mind, and the mind ultimately drives and controls the physical world. This has led to the unfortunate proposition that nothing real exists but the mind, and the mind is the creator of the universe.

The first observation to make in this regard is that no mind has been able to control death. No mind has been able to stop the various forces of time and nature from proceeding along their paths. No one's mind, despite the pitch that the mind is exceedingly powerful, has been able to avert the body's eventual death.

Furthermore, we can easily observe in our own lives and in others, that no mind has been able to control much else — outside of a limited range of control over the body's activities — when it comes to the rest of the physical world. In other words, we cannot control the weather with our minds. We cannot control earthquakes. We cannot control the rising or setting of the sun. We cannot control any of the other activities of the universe. They all proceed regardless of whether our minds try to stop them. They all manage to continue despite what we think.

The deceptive part of this very seductive proposal (that the mind is the controlling entity of the universe) is that if the mind is not in control of things around us, then the mind must secretly want those things to happen. There is some subconscious mental will going on that contradicts the conscious mind, and the universe is proceeding because of this subconscious will.

Then we must ask: why is the universe proceeding along its path of time the same way for everyone? If our mind can control the universe, then why hasn't anyone's mind been able to take control over all the hassles and struggles we face on this planet? The only logical response is that the mind cannot control the universe.

Furthermore, there are some glaring contradictions to the notion that the mind is, or could be, in control. We can simply observe one of these contradictions among the many self-help gurus that promote this concept: How is it that while the mind is supposed to be the all-pervading controller of existence, these self-help gurus must pitch us with their lectures and numerous self-help books? If they've been so successful at accomplishing their teachings, why can't they simply just *make us* better with their minds? The techniques proposed by these self-help gurus may vary slightly, but the intent of their education is generally to help their students gain greater wealth, fame, success, attention and influence by changing our thinking, and realizing that our mind is in control. If the self-help gurus' minds had such control, why couldn't they simply change our thinking directly?

The other problem with this teaching is that it assumes the person is the mind. If the person is the mind, *then who is it* that decides to *change our mind?* In order to change the mind there must be someone—a driver and observer—who can intend and initiate that change. Furthermore, as noted in these works, the process required in order to change the mind is quite difficult. *Who* is the constant force making the determination to change the mind; despite all of its former thinking habits? Lastly, *who* is remaining to reap the rewards once the mind has been changed? If the self is the mind, and the mind is changed, that former self is gone once the mind changes. Therefore, no one remains to realize any reward, since the last mind—the one who initially read the self-help guru's book—is gone, replaced by the changed mind.

What is the Mind?

Put simply, the mind is like a software program and the brain is like a computer. Computer hardware consists of wires and chips, which communicate and store information in the form of electronic on-off states—also called bits. A combination of these on-off states or bits makes up a byte. A byte is like a word and bits are like letters. A string of these bytes becomes an instruction. A group of these instructions becomes a program, and together, programs make up the software of the computer.

The actual wires and transistors of the computer (and the various other electronics such as resistors) make up the hardware of the computer—they are the solid objects, while the software is the information that instructs the hardware operations. The software will define how the hardware works, in other words.

In a computer, the software information is stored on hard diskettes located within the computer's hardware. Electromagnetic pulses are recorded onto the magnetic medium of these hard disks. This is done through a magnetizing head. Once the disk information is stored, it can be retrieved using another type of head — a magnetic reader.

The computer's operations are ultimately instructed by the operator, who sits aloof from the computer and its software. The operator utilizes the computer by staring into the computer screen while operating a keyboard and mouse. Through the screen, keyboard and mouse, the operator drives the operations of the computer. As the operator sends commands through the keyboard and mouse, the screen indicates the feedback of those instructions. Through this system, the computer will be driven to do many complicated tasks, including hunting around the world-wide web (internet) for all sorts of information, games and communications with others.

The mind's software transcends the brain and body just as the computer's software transcends the actual hard disk and other hardware of the computer. Just as the operating system software provides an interfacing language between the various hardware devices of the computer, the mind interacts closely with the limbic system and neural networks of the brain to execute commands to the body. These commands operate the body through the means of electromagnetic pulses through neurons.

These electromagnetic pulses through neurons make up a series of waveforms. A single wave could be compared to a bit, while a series of interfering waves could be compared to a software byte.

Just as the software of the computer must be instructed by an operator using commands entered through a keyboard and/or mouse, the mind is ultimately driven by the inner self. The self uses the mind to send commands through the brain's prefrontal cortex and limbic system.

The body is also rigged with sensory nerves and sensory organs. These reflect back to the mind images of the events of the body. These images include what the eyes see, what the tongue tastes, what the nose smells, what the skin touches and so on. These images are then reflected onto the 'screen' of the mind for the inner self — the operator — to perceive. Just as the computer operator looks at the computer monitor screen for input and feedback, the inner self perceives the electromagnetic images of the mindscreen for the body's sensory input and feedback.

Like the body, the mind is an instrument of the intentional self. The mind is a subtle sorting, translating and recording device. The intentional self is the driver of the mind. The mind takes in the images from the senses, and categorizes them onto its mind-brain mapping system, while the self is the viewer of the mapped images. Using these images, the inner self steers the mind — which then steers the body — in an attempt to achieve the objectives of the self. This is executed through the neural network of the body.

This means that the mind is a changeable, subtle mechanism distinct from the self. The separate existence of the mind can be easily shown in practical behavior: We can observe the mind's recording ability when a vision or piece of music can be recalled minutes, days and even years after first being sensed. After watching a movie with special effects, we can close our eyes and watch a scene's mental imprint on the mind. We can also replay music recorded by the mind. We may hum or sing the words of a song we heard previously, with the tune replaying in our mind long after the song was heard.

After we look at an image, we can close our eyes and see that same image imprinted upon the mind.

Like a television or a radio, we can also change the mind's images. We can decide to change our focus from one image to another. We can also observe how the mind can change from new images. We can watch the mind's images and see how new sensory inputs affect those images. Our mind can also associate and compare previously stored images with the incoming sensory images of tastes, sounds, tactile sensations and other images our senses collect over the years. As the mind imprints and arranges these images, the inner self subtly directs the mind to record these images, cataloging them according to priority. As these are sorted, the mind's priorities might be changed by the self. Physical reactions to those images might be rearranged —

driven by the self's response to watching the mindscreen. In other words, we can each *change our mind.*

Where is the Mind?

Western science has been struggling with the location of the mind for thousands of years. The Greek physician Galen of Pergamon (129-210 B.C.) struggled with the then-accepted *cardiocentric theory*—which proposed that the seat of the mind is in the heart. Galen produced a number of anatomical experiments with vivisection, illustrating the difference between the central nervous system and the arterial system. Despite some intense debate among the Stoics and others following Galen's experiments, there was increasing acceptance that the central nervous system played an integral role in the mind's processes. Yet from these ancient times to the modern day, researchers are still speculating and debating on the precise location of the mind.

The planaria worm (*Dugesia dorotocephala*) was Dr. James McConnell's favorite lab subject for his conditioning studies that began in 1955. In one cruel test, Dr. McConnell subjected a group of planaria to bright light followed by a mild electric shock. The shock would make the worms curl up in pain. This light-and-shock sequence was repeated hundreds of times for reinforcement. Eventually the worms would immediately curl up once the light was turned on, with or without a shock. This illustrated not only the worms' conscious attempts to avoid pain (a concept often ignored by modern science), but also their ability to remember the circumstances surrounding the pain. Where were these memories stored?

The planaria worm has a tiny brain and central nervous system, just as most humans and animals have. However, these worms have an incredible ability to reproduce immediately upon being cut or sliced. This is commonly referred to as *regeneration.* Not all sliced worms regenerate on both ends. Most will at least regenerate at the tail end. Many amphibians also have this ability—they will typically regenerate a limb following its amputation. The planarian worm, however, can be cut in half and each half will develop into a physically complete organism.

This is thought to occur through a regeneration of the head on the tail side of the split and *vice versa*. Each side then will develop a full body, tail and head.

In order to test for the location of memory, Dr. McConnell cruelly sliced the planarians into two pieces, in the middle of the body between the head and tail. Assuming memory was stored in the head end — where the central nervous system is — the head-end regeneration should remember the light-shock training and curl up. Meanwhile, the tail-end regeneration would not remember the shock treatment.

Not so fast. Contrary to this assumption, both regenerated worm halves remembered the training, and in many cases, the tail-generated worms remembered the training better than the brain-side worm did. This research theoretically indicated that memory was not necessarily stored in the brain (McConnell *et al.* 1960).

This research underscores some of the studies referenced earlier, showing continuing memory and cognition despite partial brain removal or damage to loci known for particular functions. In Mishkin (1978) and Mumby *et al.* (1992), for example, surgical removal of the amygdala and hippocampus resulted either in minor memory impairment or none at all. Vargha-Khadem and Polkey (1992) reviewed multiple studies of hemidecortication — the removal of at least half of the brain. Full cognitive recovery following hemidecortication resulted in more than 80% of all subjects.

Magnetic imaging of human patients following brain damage has confirmed the movement of mental functions from one part of the brain to the other. This has resulted in the theory of brain plasticity, as discussed earlier. It is not difficult to logically conclude that if mental function moves from one part of the brain to another, the mind must have a composition separate from the brain tissues. Truly, this composition has continued to baffle researchers. Imaging can locate electromagnetic activity indicating cognition, memory and decision-making — the executive activities — within the brain. Electromagnetic activity may also indicate active regions and pathways during particular thought activity. Yet the precise location and composition of the mind and memory has remained mysterious.

We should consider also that the brain is not restricted to the gray matter within the skull. This region of the brain is composed of the right and left hemispheres of the *cerebrum*, the *cerebellum*, and the *brain stem* — composed of the *midbrain*, the *pons* and *medulla*. Also included in the brain is the *spinal column* and *spinal nerves*. It would thus be more accurate to describe the "brain" as the *central nervous system* or the *neural network*, which expands to the *peripheral nervous system* located throughout the body. The spinal column and spinal nerve system serve as a bridge between the lower activity centers (or *chakras*) and the higher and more subtle waveform translation centers of the brain. From the spinal column radiates various waveforms that stimulate organ activity. These direct pathways from the spine drive the autonomic systems and the programmed response centers throughout the central nervous system.

The virtual link between the senses, the brain and the mind lies hidden within the waveform interference patterns guided by the self through the limbic system and imaging cortices. The inner self's executive processes are generated through the prefrontal cortex and translated through the thalamus, hypothalamus and hippocampal complex to their respective loci. These areas are considered the interbrain. Using a network of subtle and gross conduits, they negotiate the information between the senses and the subtle mind. They also bridge the feedback of the mind's instructions and the initiation of brain and motor function. For this reason, many physicians attribute the amygdala as being the seat of emotion, although removal of it does not prevent emotion to be exhibited.

Why is this? This is because emotion arises from the unseen inner self. The limbic system provides an insertion point for emotions to guide and steer the processes of prioritization. In other words, a surgeon will not find any emotion within a surgically removed limbic organ.

The neural network is a system of interconnected neurons. Connecting different parts of the anatomy are nerve tracts.

Nerve tracts are armored passageways that protect neurons and accelerate wave transmissions. These tracts might be compared to a household network of wire conduits protecting the wires and circuitry. When electricity must travel through underground wires, heavy-duty conduit piping will be used as shielding. These pipe tubes protect the wires from the decomposing elements of the soil. They also protect the local environment from electricity running through the wiring.

Nerve tracts serve similar purposes within the body. They provide the sheathing allowing pulsed waveforms to channel throughout the body. They also conduct and direct informational pulses to specific locations around the body.

The intentional reflections of the self are translated through the mind into physiological instructions. Once translated, they will stimulate both the motor cortex and the thalamus and hypothalamus. The thalamus regulates or adjusts thermogenesis, which controls the body's heat levels, providing a foundation for metabolic activity. Meanwhile the hypothalamus negotiates the sympathetic and parasympathetic activities of the body's autonomic system through the stimulation of the pituitary gland. Via the hypothalamus, the mind dictates control to regulate the functions of the body's metabolic activities through the pathways of the endocrine system.

Through the vehicle of the motor cortex, the mind stimulates physical activity. We can thus conclude from these basic physiological cascades—confirmed by many years of research—that the physical interface or conduit between the mind and the physical body is located in the limbic system. This might be compared to the magnetic heads that 'read' the polarity states recorded onto a computer's hard disks.

The cascade of signals from the limbic system is also regulated by the activities of the pineal gland, which coordinate with the rhythmic SCN cells to secrete melatonin. Melatonin triggers a cascading pathway to slow metabolism, leading to sleep and cell repair. Melatonin levels are balanced by other metabolic biochemicals stimulated through other command cascades. Examples of these are cortisol and the thyroid hormones.

All of these physical components of the brain and signaling systems fall within the perimeter of the mind. The brain is a physical transfer and conversion mechanism. The mind is a holographic echoing mechanism utilizing interference patterns and standing waveforms to play out the intentions of the self.

Dr. Jim Tucker, a professor at the University of Virginia, compares the mind's relationship with the brain and body to a television set (2005). Dr. Tucker explains that while the TV signal is translated through the television set, the signal of television programming originates from a remote location. In the same way, Dr. Tucker explains, the mind is not the brain, but rather, he insists, the signals of the mind are transmitted through the brain.

The neurological research headed up by Dr. Robert Knight illustrated that brainwaves allow regions of the brain to communicate using combinations of interactive alpha, beta, gamma and theta waves. According to the research, the synchronization or *coupling* effect of these various waves—together with their timing and frequency—transmit specific information. We can certainly compare the television and television programming—like the computer and computer software—to the brain and the mind. However, the transfer of the information occurs in precisely the same fashion in all of these cases: Through waveform interference pattern transmission.

This all implies the use of a subtle conscious sorting process. When we consider computer memory, for example, data is not being recorded onto silicon. Silicon is acting as a *conductor* for the arrangements of 0s and 1s. These assembled messages are magnetically recorded onto a hard drive tape or disk. If we were to remove that hard drive from the computer and look at it, we will not see any data. We might see a tiny round disk inside of the drive case—like a miniature CD. If we pulled out the disk from the case and looked at it, we still would not see any information. This is because the information is magnetically stored onto the surface of the disk.

Hard drive disks are coated with a metal alloy like iron oxide or cobalt alloy. The surface is divided into tiny magnetic regions, each separated to enable a polarizing of the molecules on the surface of the disk. A single polar magnetized molecule contains no information in itself. Nor is the information contained on the magnetic reader. The combinations of polarity contain the message, which are meaningless until they are compiled and converted by the software. These on or off *permutations* must first be arranged into a sequence code into machine code by a translation program in the CPU. This code is then translated into operating system instructions that feed information back to the operator via the monitor.

In the same way, although the physical anatomy of brain gyrus, neurons and the various organs of the limbic system appear to contain the information and memory that resonates through them, they are no more containing our memories than the metal computer box contains any data. Informational waveforms resonate *through* the neurons, where they are crystallized, translated and broadcast into the neural net: It is the translation of the waveform interference patterns that creates the information.

The complex exchange of instantaneous waveform pulses moving through the body is nothing short of astounding. Some estimate that over six trillion waveform messages per minute are fired through the nervous system alone—not including the higher frequency microtubule pulses, the various hormone releases, the intercellular biocommunication and the intracellular network. These waveforms pulsing through the physical layers are all sorted for priority and projected through the mind to be imaged by the self.

Research has illustrated that the left side of the brain is associated with the thoughts relating to logic, language, and mathematics. Meanwhile the right side of the brain has been associated with art, fantasy, and music. Further to this point of specialization, certain regions appear to associate with certain mental skills and particular types of memories. Auditory communication, for example, is associated with the temporal lobe, while written motor skills have been linked with the motor cortex of the frontal lobe. Visual interaction usually utilizes the occipital lobe. Recent neurological research has confirmed that each of these brain functions also run concurrent with particular types of brainwaves. We also know a hierarchy of waveforms is slated to each thought-type. The slower waves like delta and theta tend to accompany sleep and introspection, while faster waves like beta and gamma waves tend to accompany sensual cognition and information transfer.

This indicates that the inner self's intentions are expressed through the mind and brain via these brain waveforms. We can see this should we gather various opinions from people. While a group of people may receive the same information through the senses, a variety of perceptions and conclusions will be made by each. Even though the mind may meticulously gather incoming sensory information, the unique self can shape and prioritize this information through intention.

Scientific research confirms that information is sorted, prioritized, organized and prepared for storage after input from the sensory system. Research illustrates that the visual cortex will shape and direct spatial visual information as it is being gathered through signaling mechanisms. This process has been termed *retino-cortical mapping* (Johnston 1986).

The entire process of the brain and central nervous system would be impossible without an operator and a power supply driving the sorting operations of the mind. At the end of the day, the self is the operator. The mind is the software and the brain is the CPU. The body is the hardware.

Mind Science

The modern western notions of psychology and mental health as we know them today have been only recently developed. In the middle ages, a religious fanaticism took hold of Europe, which led to the widespread belief that mental disease was the result of demonic possession. The ancient sciences had a much more logical and realistic vision of the mind and the self.

Psychology and psychiatry is thought to have arose only during the late nineteenth century (as through humankind were Neanderthals prior to that): A limited view to say the least.

Wilhelm Wundt is thus considered the father of modern psychology. He founded a laboratory in 1879 at the University of Leipzig — where he was a professor. Two years later, he founded the first European psychology journal, and wrote a number of books on the subject. Professor Wundt's *structuralism* model of the mind proposed the dividing of the mind into various parts, with each part performing different tasks. This theory later gave way to the modern theories of *functionalism* and *behaviorism*.

Unbeknownst to Wundt, the role of the unconscious mind had been studied for thousands of years. The Greeks were known to use hypnosis, and they studied the undercurrent of the mind together with the dreamscape. The art of hypnosis was somewhat lost, however, until it was revived by Franz Mesmer in the eighteenth century. Mesmer's proposal was that hypnosis was created by a force of nature called *animal magnetism,* which seemingly overwhelmed his subjects as they encountered magnets — adjusting the body's tidal influences. Interestingly, Mesmer also proposed that life moves through the body via thousands of tiny channels. The flow of life through these channels, he thought, was subject to various environmental influences, including spiritual forces and the movement of planets. One might wonder whether Mesmer studied the ancient Ayurvedic and/or Chinese systems. Nonetheless, hypnotism became controversial to say the least.

It was not until Scottish surgeon James Braid announced that hypnotism was genuine in the 1840s that hypnotism was accepted as anything other than a form of hysteria in Europe and America. Hypnosis was largely overlooked during the years following. Its use as a form of treatment only became more prominent in the late nineteenth century and the early twentieth century. Today hypnosis is accepted and widely used by many researchers, psychologists, and psychiatrists.

The concept that prevailed in the nineteenth century was one describing the mind as consisting of different levels of consciousness. A number of theories were proposed on the nature and functions of these portions. Probably the most famous were those of Dr. Pierre Marie Félix Janet and Dr. Sigmund Freud, both prominent psychologists during the late nineteenth and early twentieth centuries. Janet is attributed to have arrived at the theory of the mind being divided into *conscious, unconscious* and *preconscious* parts. In the 1920s, Freud proposed the mind contained three different components: the *ego*, the *super-ego* and the *id*. Freud's theory took center stage as a possible explanation of various behavioral problems confronting physicians and psychologists since that time.

Both Freud and Janet gathered a great deal of information through hypnotism. By hypnotizing people, Freud and Janet *regressed* them to re-experience the behavior or thinking that occurred prior to a current disorder. Though many insights and disease pathologies came out of this research, it was generally regarded as having fallen short of proving the existence of the three parts of the mind.

The proposal regarding mental disease stemming from the three sections of the mind was rooted in the assumption that the mind is constantly in conflict. Freud proposed that a conflict between these three parts of the mind creates mental disturbance, while a balance between them creates mental health. He proposed that the *id* is the unconscious source encouraging the gratification of desires, rooted in the most basic desires of survival. Meanwhile the *super-ego* was supposed to have been in opposition with these desires, acting as the conscience.

According to Freud's theories, the *ego* supposedly mediates between the *id* and *super-ego*, presenting the conscious portion of the mind to the world. The science of psychology has accepted the assumption of a conscious and subconscious apportionment of the mind. However, various ancillary theories have been presented over the years since Janet and Freud.

Unsatisfied with the ability to change a person's behavior using hypnotism, Janet and Freud embarked on their now-famous methods of *psychoanalysis*. These methods are still used today by psychologists and psychiatrists, and are actually quite basic: The patient is simply encouraged to discuss problems and issues the patient feels is related to the dilemma at hand.

The method of hypnosis in psychiatric treatment is based upon the use of *autosuggestion*. The process usually begins with the hypnotist positioning before the patient and suggesting the patient is becoming sleepy and relaxed. Sometimes distractive rhythmic devices are used, the most famous of which is a small pendulum. As the trust in the hypnotist develops within the patient, the patient dozes off into a state of *suggestibility*—being open to suggestion. During this time, the patient may be clearly aware of the events transpiring—or not, depending upon the suggestions of the hypnotist. Depending upon the type of hypnosis given, the patient may also be drawn into a deeper state where the patient may not be able to recall the hypnosis episode consciously. This has often been described as an altered state of consciousness.

One discipline, which has its roots in Freud's use of hypnotism, is *autogenics*, introduced by Dr. Malcolm Caruthers in the 1970s. The word autogenic refers to something generated from within. The *autogenic training system* consists of becoming aware of the body's autonomic nervous system, and being able to control both sympathetic and parasympathetic physical responses to stress. This was accomplished primarily through visualization techniques.

Another important psychological system, also deeply steeped in the concepts of the conscious and unconscious mind, is behaviorism. Research into behavior modification was made famous by the work of Ivan Pavlov, who in the early twentieth century worked with both animals and humans to understand how the mind can connect pleasure and pain with particular *triggers*, which bring about a trained response. The cruel dog-salivation experiments of Pavlov's dog experiments are quite famous, and they have given birth to a number of behavioral psychological theories and practices. One of the more notable behavioral theorists is B. F. Skinner. Professor Skinner's research into conditioning and behavior modification has become a foundation for many of the psychological theories assumed today.

A distant relative of behaviorism is functionalism. This concept was advanced by Dr. Alan Turing. In 1950, Dr. Turing laid out the fundamentals of the theory with his article *Computing Machinery and Intelligence.* Dr. Turing proposed that the mind is a learning machine of sorts, accumulating experience throughout ones lifetime.

Of course, behavior modification and conditioning — or *operant conditioning* — has been commonly used by parents, teachers and authoritarians over the duration of human existence. This system is also embedded into the natural world. It is not hard to observe that as we experience events and the consequences of our actions, we begin to learn that certain activities have better results than do others. This realization theoretically changes our behavior, leading to a gradual process of evolution. Those who do not adjust their behavior or learn the lessons, on the other hand, are destined to face a recurrence of those lessons until they are learned.

After many years of hypnotherapy, the fundamental mechanisms — along with the supposed conscious and unconscious mind themselves — are still considered mysterious by western science. Some propose suggestibility is simply a state of mind and hypnosis is simply the succumbing to suggestion. However, there is enough documented evidence of hypnotized patients retrieving historical information not accessible when conscious to consider the alternatives. This lends credence to the position of the mind held by the ancient sciences.

The Mind-Brain Bridge

Over the past couple of decades, the study of the mind has been directed towards the electromagnetic properties of the brain's neurons. This trend towards a physiological interpretation of the mind through the transduction of electrical activity between neurons necessitates the assumption that the mind and brain are one and the same.

The primary means for research promoting this assumption has been the use of various radiative imaging systems such as EEG (electroencephalography), MEG (magneto encephalography), MRI (magnetic resonance imagery), PET (positron emission tomography), and CAT (computer-aided tomography).

These imaging systems each focus on different waveform attributes of brain neurons, as they are altered by these different forms of radiation.

These imaging devices have determined that the bridge between the mind and the brain are distinct electromagnetic waveforms called brainwaves.

The notion that the mind and the brain were connected through electromagnetic brainwaves has developed over the past century. The mapping of the brain using electricity was pioneered during the 1920s by Dr. Wilder Penfield, who touched various parts of subjects' brains with electrode sensors while they lay conscious on the operating table prior to or following brain surgery. Dr. Penfield began noticing commonalities between patient responses as he touched certain parts of the brain. Dr. Penfield accumulated enough data over time to develop a map of the various cortex regions and sensory regions. Dr. Penfield co-authored the landmark *Epilepsy and the Functional Anatomy of the Human Brain* (1951) with Dr. Herbert Jasper, a reference still used today.

Dr. Penfield's research focused on epileptics initially. He observed that regional brain activity was relative to types of thoughts, memories, and activity. Dr. Penfield found that if he stimulated a part of the brain with the electrode, he could provoke a particular type of memory. This led to Dr. Penfield and the rest of the medical community surmising that memory is retained within particular specialized brain cells within certain regions. Furthermore, he concluded that particular parts of the brain specialized in certain types of thoughts or activities. The subsequent mapping not only identified functional parts of the brain. It also identified which types of memories were theoretically stored within that particular region. These mapped locations were called *engrams.*

In the 1940s, a psychologist named Dr. Karl Lashley conducted cruel research that contradicted this notion that memories were located in specific brain neurons. Dr. Lashley trained mice to particular tasks and then cruelly removed different parts of their brains. He then reintroduced the mice to the same circumstances, and found that despite brain cell areas associated with those memories being removed, they were still able to remember the tasks learned prior to the surgery. Furthermore, even when most of the rats' brains were removed, the rats were unexpectedly still able to remember what was taught to them prior to the surgery.

A prominent neuroscientist, Dr. Karl Pribran, followed this research with many years of study on memory and engrams. Dr. Pribran's initial research focused on the frontal cortex of monkeys and cats, and his research identified specific areas of the brain associated with particular cognitive functions. However, he was intrigued by repeated results—like Dr. Lashley—indicating that when specific neurons or regions were removed or severed, cognition predominantly continued. For example, he found that an image could still be perceived in detail when the optic nerve was severed. This led to Dr. Pribran's conclusion that perception and cognition went deeper than the brain's anatomy.

Years earlier, Dr. Lashley had entertained the notion of a wave interference pattern for memories. Dr. Pribran worked closely with renowned physicists Dr. David Bohm and Dr. Dennis Gabor—the 1971 physics Nobel laureate. Together they arrived at the notion that cognition and memory were related to the mechanics of wave transmission. Using *Fourier analysis*—in which sine wave function is calculated within the context of the action, the *holonomic brain model of cognitive function* was born. This theory was proposed along the lines of the *Gabor function*, which was put forth by Dr. Gabor to propose the natural existence of the hologram (Pribran 1991).

When we examine some of the expansive research done in the field of brainwaves, we see how both brain function and the mind are closely related to wave mechanics. The electroencephalogram measures the voltage potential differences among different regions of the brain. These voltage differences result in a wave formation, which can range in wavelength, frequency and amplitude among a collection of neurons. These brainwaves are not single units in themselves. They are surges of collective interference patterns created by the electrical pulses of neurons throughout the body.

Delta brainwaves cycle from one to three hertz, and tend to predominate during NREM (non-rapid eye movement) sleep, and some meditation. During this type of sleep, dreaming is minimal and the body is often in motion. Delta waves tend to resonate more actively in the frontal cortex. Delta waves correlate with an increase in the production and circulation of growth hormone. One of growth hormone's more important attributes within the body is its ability to advance the healing and regeneration process while our body is sleeping.

Theta brainwaves cycle at four to seven hertz and dominate during mid-stage sleeping. Theta waves are more elusive, but seem to most active during memory retrieval and consolidation during sleep, and become more active in creative endeavors and behavior modification during waking hours. The hippocampus appears to actively accommodate and transduce these waves. Observations have noted peak hippocampus activity during predominantly theta wave periods. The hippocampus is associated with spatial recognition and short-term memory consolidation.

Alpha brainwaves will cycle at eight to thirteen cycles per second, and are dominant during light sleep and dreaming, as well as some meditation states. Alpha waves are seen dominant during memorization tasks, especially those related to words, persons and visual impressions.

Beta brainwaves will cycle at fourteen to thirty hertz and are dominant during active, waking consciousness. These waves tend to be prominent towards the front of the brain on the side predominating during that activity. Beta waves reflect a state of focused attention and activity. A lack of beta waves during waking hours — or lower frequency beta waves — tends to occur with a lack of focus or concentration. On the other hand, as brainwave levels increase toward the higher range of beta and into the gamma range at over thirty cycles per second, a higher level of mental focus occurs.

Gamma brainwaves are higher frequency brain waves, and are often referred to as high-frequency beta waves. Gamma waves predominate during intense problem solving and focused learning. Gamma waves cycle at thirty to sixty hertz. Recent research has determined that gamma waves will be synchronized and coded by phase within the visual cortex. This phase shifting creates a coherence mechanism—a sorting process where gamma waves with the same phases are segregated and commingled. The resulting sorting process allows the gamma waves to interfere and provide associations of particular thoughts, images or impressions of sensual information.

High gamma brainwaves cycle from sixty to two hundred hertz, and have only become obvious to researchers using more sensitive equipment. These brainwaves are seen during the most intense cognitive functions. The slower waves of theta, delta and alpha tend to resonate with distinct physical attributes. The high gamma waves tend to relate to higher states, and tend to be more diverse in their connection points around the regions of the central nervous system. In one study of eight subjects, for example, high gamma brainwave activity increased during the practice of *pranayama*—a method of concentrated meditative breath control (Vialatte *et al.* 2008).

Another type of brainwave found by researchers are called *ripples*. Ripples are high frequency oscillations that appear to be generated in the hippocampus. They have been observed oscillating with the negative portion of slower brainwaves. Ripples appear to transduce through the medial temporal lobe, notably between the hippocampus and the rhinal cortex—a region associated with the processing of explicit memory recall. Explicit memory includes active intentional recall during conscious cognition. In other words, ripples appear to function as informational waveform 'bites' used to access recent, conscious memories and instructions. They are part of our active information biocommunication system.

The discovery of ripples augments our position that EEG research has tended to oversimplify the role of brain waveforms that oscillate through the various neurons. The brain's mapping has focused on larger regions of the brain. There are still intra-neuronal networks that function on a more subtle basis.

For example, a central pivoting exchange factor of the brain's networking system includes the *pyramidal neuron networks*. Pyramidal neurons lie within the cortex regions of the brain. Regions more dense with pyramidal neurons are often collectively referred to as the *neocortex*. Here their densities can be as high as 75%. Researchers have estimated the total number of pyramidal neurons in the brain to be in the neighborhood of fifteen to twenty billion. These specialized neurons crystallize and transduce waveform signals between the cortices and the rest of the central nervous system.

Some of these signals have different frequency attributes. They appear to transduce through the polar gateway systems of ion channels. These are not unlike the on-off states of computer machine code, except there is typically more than one type of on-off state among each gateway, to allow for feedback loops. Another, more dimensional description of this transduction is called *signal coupling*. This is when multiple waveforms are "coupled" to create a unique pattern. We might refer to this as a *multiple wave interference model*.

Research has clocked the brain's activity at speeds of between 1/1000 and 10/1000 of a second, which would convert to 100-1000 meters/second. As these frequencies relate to the wave nature of the electrical activity of the brain, they also imply that there is a rhythmic function to the mechanics of the mind. The fact that the frequency increases as our mind becomes more active indicates that higher activity exerts a greater wave speed.

Certainly if we consider how instantaneous reactions and thoughts move around the body, we are talking not only about speed. We are dealing with a network broadcasting system allowing nearly instantaneous communication. This communication system is linear yet still global: concurrently spreading through the neurons and tissues into the vast territory of organs, tissues and muscles. This might be best compared to the network access of a website to billions of browsers connected on the internet.

These pathways for waveform broadcasting also bridge with the mind to form complete images. Multiple researchers have confirmed that neurons of the visual cortex do not readily pick the full spectrum of frequencies necessary to form a complete image of what we perceive. The ramification of this is significant: We typically assume that what we perceive is "out there" in the physical domain. We assume that we are receiving a complete picture. Rather, we are perceiving a combination of what our senses take in and what our mind extrapolates.

Illustrating this, Russian scientist Dr. Nikolai Bernstein performed film studies on human perception for several decades in the mid-twentieth century. His research showed that human movement could be translated into wave patterns using Fourier calculations.

This is confirmed as we watch television or a movie. When we perceive movement on the TV or movie screen, we are not actually seeing movement among the screen images. We are merely seeing a series of still pictures flashed in sequence faster than we can perceive. Between the flashed images is a significant dead space or dark image. Our minds fill in the blanks and create the illusion of movement.

The work of neuroscientist Dr. Russell DeValois focused on this element of visual perception over the past several of decades. His research papers documented how the mind integrates batches of visual inputs such as color and motion. His years of groundbreaking research culminated in the 1990 compendium *Spatial Vision*, co-authored with his wife Kathleen—also a professor in the subject. His memorial quoted him describing his lifetime's work in visual perception as, *"the physiological and anatomical organization underlying visual perception. In particular, how wavelength information is analyzed and encoded, the contribution of wavelength and luminance information to spatial vision, and how spatial information is analyzed and encoded in the visual nervous system."*

In one study performed by Dr. DeValois at the University of California at Berkeley, the responses of cats and monkeys were analyzed while responding to visual checkerboard patterns. Rather than responding to the patterns themselves, the animals

responded to the interference patterns created by the complementary aspects of the design—consistent with Fourier-calcu-
lated interference waves.

The work of Dr. Fergus Campbell at Cambridge University
has confirmed that the human cerebral cortex picks up particular
frequencies and not others. The cerebral component neurons are
'tuned' to specific wavelengths and frequencies. Dr. Pribran also
confirmed this in his sometimes-cruel studies on cats and monkeys. During these tests, it became apparent that combinations of
waves of particular frequencies were being received, processed
and converted into perceived images as they were combined
with internally created waveforms. These internal waveforms
are drawn from memory through a hierarchical cortical mapping
sorting process.

In the 1970s, Dr. Benjamin Libet began researching decision-
making and brain electrical response at the University of California at San Francisco. His goal was to explore a concept first
introduced by Luder Deeke and Hans Kurnhuber called
bereitschafts-potential – which translates to *readiness potential*. In
Dr. Libet's studies, human volunteers hooked up to an electro-
encephalograph were told to perform activities such as button
pressing or finger flicking. Dr. Libet's research compared three
points in time: When the subject consciously made the decision
to press the button; when the button was pressed; and when
brainwaves indicated an instruction from the motor cortex was
made using the EEG. As expected, the conscious decision preceded the button pushing by an average of about 200 milliseconds (or 150 milliseconds considering a 50 msec margin of
error).

Surprisingly, however, the brainwaves associated with the
instruction to press the bottom actually preceded the subject's
conscious decision to take the action. Stunned by these results,
Dr. Libet and others spent several years confirming the results.
Several scientific articles documented the findings (Libet *et al.*
1983; Libet 1985). These results indicated that the action somehow was not originating from the conscious mind, but must be
coming from a deeper source.

Still, as Dr. Libet wrote in 2003, the gap between the conscious mind and the physical act gives the conscious mind an ability to *"block or veto the process, resulting in no motor act."* This, Dr. Libet said, is confirmed by the common experience of consciously blocking urges incompatible with social acceptability.

In 2004 — more than two decades after his groundbreaking discovery — Dr. Libet proposed a theory based on his and others' research in this area. He called this the *conscious mental field theory*. This theory proposed that the mind is a sphere of activity bridging the pulsing of nerve cells with the subjective conscious experience. He described this subjective experience as an outgrowth of the various pulses — a sort of gathering or convergence of various inputs.

A neuron is made up of a cell body with a nucleus, and two types of nerve fibers that extend outward from the cell body. The fibers include *dendrites,* which conduct informational waveforms into the neural cell body. *Axons,* on the other hand, project waveforms outward, away from the cell body. Most neurons have multiple dendrites that spider outward making several connections. Sensory nerves typically have only one dendrite, however. Sensory nerves are also typically longer — sometimes measuring up to a meter in length. Dendrites act as receptors. They are tuned into the pulsed waveform messages that pass from neuron to neuron. They carry this rhythmic information into the neuron cell body where it may be translated or even transmuted before being conducted or broadcasted. In some cases, the neuron may simply conduct and amplify the waveform.

In addition to specialized sensory neurons referred to as *afferent nerves,* there are also motor neurons, which are usually referred to as *efferent neurons.* The efferent or motor neurons are designed to carry instructional waveforms outward through the central nervous system to specific skeletal or organ cells. In these locations, these cells respond as instructed by the information provided by these waveform interference patterns. We note this because a single waveform does not necessarily contain enough information to drive a complex motor process. It takes a waveform combination to affect these specialized cells. Some are stimulated into metabolism responses, secretions, or contractions. Because they are stimulated by the efferent neurons, these cells are called *effectors.*

The inner self ultimately stimulates the effector neurons through the facilities offered by the neural network. The neural network generally has three basic types of processes: The first is to receive and translate afferent sensory waveforms from the senses and environment. The second is to project instructional waveform combinations outward through the appropriate neural tracts. The third process of the neural net is to prioritize, sort and catalog memories and various autonomic programs.

The brain grows and develops in the body from a tubular canal called the *neural tube.* The entire brain is made up of billions of neurons. These are networked into bundles of groupings, which include *nerve tracts, gyri, fissures, sulci* and *cerebrum lobes.* These groupings of specialized neurons work conjunctively to accomplish specialized tasks, while transmitting information back and forth through neural superhighways. The locations of these nerve groupings will be common. Most nerve functions thus have *location plasticity.* Plasticity is the ability of the organism to move or reorganize the location or processes involved in accomplishing particular tasks. In other words, should one location not be able to function, the organism will relocate the function to another region of the brain.

The inner self steers the neural network through the frontal cortex. Here the various waveforms provided by the senses and the body's feedback are observed by the self. The inner self utilizes the command center of the prefrontal cortex to respond to these images. This is located towards the front of the brain, behind and on top of the forehead.

This prefrontal and frontal cortex region provides the gateway for the inner self to not only observe the condition of the body and the environment, but also submit executive orders through the mind in response. Subsequently, brain researchers have determined that the frontal lobes are stimulated during the processing of decisions related to right and wrong, the prioritization of consequences, and logical thinking. Through the prefrontal region, the self expresses personality and submits executive orders.

The *motor cortex* lies just behind the frontal cortex as we comb back over the head on each side. The motor cortex resides within a band of neural grey matter (neuron cells) that wrap around the top of the head on the left and right hemispheres. Here instructions are conducted through the frontal cortex and continue a path towards execution. Within the motor cortex reside specialized networks of neurons. Each network coordinates with specific types of motor activity and different aspects of metabolism.

The *premotor* region contains billions of specialized *mirroring* neurons, which reflect and stack the executive decisions transmitted from the frontal cortex. Behind the premotor cortex is the *primary motor cortex*. This region contains specialized neurons able to broadcast specific signals through the neural network to targeted areas of the body. One group of neurons will submit instructions to the toes, while another will submit to the feet, and so on. This organized vertical arrangement of specialized motor neurons is also referred to as the *homunculus motor* region, because each neuron group is connected to different locations around the body.

While most people have similar homunculus mapping systems, use the same regions, these motor regions of the brain also have a significant potential for plasticity. In other words, should one region of the cortex become damaged or insufficient, another set of neurons located elsewhere may take over those signaling activities. This indicates that the brain is a flexible tool for the inner self. The person is not the brain or the mind. The person is the inner operator who is directing the use of the mind and brain through the facilities offered by the neural network.

Behind the region of the motor cortex is another brain region called the *sensory cortex*. The motor cortex has several individual cortices, and spreads from the top of the head (*parietal lobe*) through the back of the head (*occipital lobe*) and along the sides (*temporal lobe*). Among these lobes lie the *visual cortex*, the *audi-*

tory cortex, the *olfactory cortex,* the *postcentral gyrus,* and the *gustatory cortex.*

In these respective regions, incoming sensory signals are translated and processed. The first three cortices — the visual, auditory and olfactory — are the centers that process the signals connected to seeing, hearing and smelling, respectively. The postcentral gyrus processes the sensory signals connected to touch and balance, while the gustatory cortex processes taste signals from the tongue. Into each sensory cortex, specialized neural tracts conduct in and blend waveforms from the sense organs. The interference patterns of these waveforms blend together to provide a compiled image for the self to observe.

The limbic system is positioned inside these cortex regions, towards the center of the brain. The limbic system is made up of the thalamus, the hypothalamus, the hippocampus, the cingulates, the fomix and the amygdala. Each of these has a slightly different function, but together they translate waveform data from the body to observations and memories for the inner self to perceive. The limbic system's role is to prioritize and sort this information according to the intentions of the self.

The hypothalamus and thalamus are the central translation system for waveforms traveling between the brain and the rest of the body. They also stimulate endocrine release of hormones and neurotransmitters, and translate incoming communications from around the body.

The cingulates are programmed to govern the autonomic systems such as the heartbeat, breathing, hunger, and so on. The amygdala, on the other hand, provides a gateway to the lower neural centers, channeling the self's focus upon survival into fear, anger and other emotions. The hippocampus then sorts and stacks all this information for memory storage.

The fomix channels the waveform information from the hippocampus through a circuitry of memory processing called the *Papex circuit.* Together the limbic system provides a translation and staging service for waveform information.

We might compare the limbic system to a computer's operating system. The software might be stored in a particular location within the computer. Nevertheless, its programming instructions govern information translation, assembly, prioritization, storage, and transmission out to the computer's peripheral systems.

The brain receives several types of input. The first is called *exteroception,* which means information gathered by the five basic senses of hearing, taste, smell, vision and touch. *Interoception* is the reception of signals received by the internal neurons, such as pain and other feedback responses. The third reception type is *proprioception,* which is the internal feedback mechanism gauging coordinated movements, balance and motor efficiency — often referred to as *kinesthesia.* Meanwhile *equilibrioception* is the feedback of motor balance information, which is coordinated with signals passing through the vestibular system. *Nociception* is the reception of pain signals that accompany a threat of damage to tissues or cells. Finally, *thermoception* is the sensing of heat or coldness within the body. Other interoceptions include the sense of time, the esophageal senses and others. A few other sensations have been proposed, though most could also be considered a subset of interoception.

Each of these types of signals is associated with a particular region of the brain — though most interact in one respect or another within the limbic system and its components. For example, proprioception appears to be stimulated within the cerebellum. Thermoception seems to propagate from thermoceptor cells in the hypothalamus. Nociception is thought to be stimulated through the *anterior cingulated gyrus* (part of the cingulates).

As waveforms are stepped up through neural tracts toward the brain, they are boosted or converted by neural gateways into waveform configurations that can be managed by the limbic system. It is through the limbic system that various cortex regions are fed interoception from around the body. Programming sequences drive autonomic responses from the cortices primarily via the limbic system as well. As waveforms travel through the limbic system, the amygdale — channeling survival concerns of the self — is able to interact and alter these waveforms on their route to the particular cortex.

This emotional interference system also works in reverse. Even if a particular decision is being channeled from the motor cortex to initiate a particular response in the body, the amygdale can alter or influence that signal, initiated primarily through the hypothalamus-pituitary pathway. As it moves back through the limbic system on its way out to stimulate particular motor nerve centers and endocrine responses, motor responses may be exaggerated or muted by fear or other emotional responses directed by the inner self.

Research has demonstrated an ion channel-based electro-chemical *beta-adrenergic modulation* (Strange and Dolan 2006) facility within the amygdale. This modulation process requires a sophisticated level of waveform collaboration between the sensual inputs coming from the cortices and those arising from the mind web. As mentioned, the amygdale sorts images or impressions to emotional criteria. This provides a stacking of the information by priority. By pegging information with emotional criteria, greater memory recall is established — as compared to images without emotional tags (Dolcos *et al.* 2006).

This blending and transduction system could be compared to the internet or worldwide web. The internet or 'web' accomplishes a peer-accepted platform for the convergence of a variety of information gateways — or website portals. The convergence of all these website portals through the internet platform allows a particular user with a computer to choose to view any of the information portals. On the internet, the computer operator can choose to view a sorted compilation of websites through a search engine. The search terms are decided upon by the viewer and computer operator.

In the case of the mind's web, the viewer and operator is the inner self. The gateways are the various pathways for waveform information being received and retained by the billions of brain cells. The limbic system offers to the inner self a platform where these information signals can be sorted and compiled.

The inner self uses the sorting facility of the mind to program the search terms and the priorities for search compilation. Once a search string is established in acquisition mode, the limbic system coordinates a search through the various neuron gateways to locate waveform information with particular specifications.

The hippocampus is a central locator and search center to the mind's web. We might compare it to the placement of information throughout a hard disk, or even the assembly of information by search engine spiders. Located on each side of the brain, in the temporal lobes, information from the senses and the body are converted by the hippocampus through a complex staging process.

As was first published in a 1957 report by Scoville and Milner and later confirmed by Squire *et al.* (1991) along with other researchers, when the hippocampus becomes damaged, the first symptom is typically disorientation, memory acquisition loss, and recall deficiency. This is also evidenced in cases of encephalitis, where the hippocampus does not receive enough oxygen. When the hippocampus is damaged, new memories cannot be retained or recalled.

The Papex circuit can be likened to the cochlear passageway that stages and converts air pressure waves into electromagnetic nerve pulses. In the hippocampal pathway, waveforms from the cortical field (*entohinal cortex, perihinal cortex, cerebral cortex*, and so on), the subcortical field (*amygdale, broca, claustrum, substantia innominata*, and so on) mix with pulses from the thalamus and hypothalamus. These pulses are channeled through the *perforant path* consisting of three regions of the *dentate gyrus*. The signals pass through the CA3 and CA1 regions and on to the *subiculum* and *parahippocampal gyrus*.

Here, between the subiculum and the parahippocampal gyrus, information in the form of interference waveform patterns is processed and translated to higher frequency waveforms — and broadcast into the neural net for storage or processing. In all, this circuit vets, tags and prioritizes information, preparing it to be cataloged. The various regions of the brain located during this search identify potential storage locations for the information. In this way, the neural regions of the brain are mapped for information storage and memory recall.

In the pathway for visual impressions, for example, wave-form combinations of different frequencies strike the retina and pass through the LGM to the visual cortex. Here in the cortex, waveforms drawn from memory through the amygdale are combined with internal stimuli waveforms and LGM waveform data to create waveform interference patterns. These interference patterns create the specific information images for the self to observe.

We might compare this with creating an image by blending pixels of different colors onto a dark screen. This is the technology computers use to display graphics. Alone each pixel does not create much of an image, but together the pixels can create a complete image on the screen.

The images the inner self observes within the cortex are thus altered by context and history. The waveforms from the amygdale and memory alter the interference patterns. This accounts for the expression that we 'see what we want to see.' The interference patterns from these different sources eventually deliver convincing impressions to the hippocampus. Because the cortex combines all these waveforms together, the waveform information is forever altered. This creates the reality that each of us perceives a slightly different picture of the world around us.

In order to attempt to 'standardize' our perception, the inner self will seek confirmation from others in the physical world. Information is thus gathered through conversation and the different forms of media. This creates a feedback loop between the amygdale, the hippocampus, and the cortices to constantly adjust our perception of reality towards the apparent perception of others. This is an intentional process because the inner self is constantly seeking affirmation from others in a never-ending quest for love and acceptance.

Mapped brain regions also sort and translate incoming waveforms from the hippocampus. These are ultimately governed and coordinated by the prefrontal cortex. The intentions of the inner self stimulate a form of waveform programming that modulates neuron channels for particular response. This creates a sorting system among those programmed neurons. The ion channel gateway states and neurotransmitter fluid content around the neuron are manipulated by the executive initiatives programmed by the mind – driven by the intentions of the self. Many pre-programmed responses are crystallized within our static DNA. Still, neurons accommodate the executive authority of the inner self, expressed and translated through the prefrontal cortex and communicated via neural pathways.

Within the limbic system, waveforms from all over the body are converged and translated together with remodeled waves from the sensory cortices and the various feedback centers throughout the body. After translation, the limbic system coordinates the instructions sent out to the body.

These are mirrored by the broadcasting of reflective signals back to the frontal cortex for executive review. Should the self respond to these inputs, executive signals are again fed back to the body through the limbic system and the motor cortex.

Here again the limbic system is acting as a transfer station, stimulating the release of various hormones through the hypothalamus and pituitary gland. These hormones cascade through the various glands of the endocrine system. This system provides the feedback pathways for executive instruction that Dr. Libet's research illustrated. The sum of the process allows conscious processing of input and feedback through nerve systems pre-programmed by the mind.

Ultimately, it is the inner self – utilizing the various equipment of the brain – who initiates executive action. Once converted through the prefrontal and frontal cortices, this is accomplished directly through executive stimulation of the motor cortex and limbic system. This is like a car driver who sets up the proper cruise control speed, then removes his foot from the gas pedal. The cruise control will maintain the speed of the car by accelerating up hills and decelerating down hills automatically. However, should the driver decide to change speeds, avert running into the car ahead, or even stop the car, the driver can immediately take over the gas pedal and control the car's speed directly.

In the same way, the self is driving the vehicle of the body through both autonomic programming and executive control. Most autonomic functions can be manipulated directly should the self consciously intend to change them. In some cases, this takes practice, as biofeedback research illustrates. This conscious insertion of executive command can be initiated even during an autonomic response, just as the car driver can hit the gas pedal at any time to change the car's speed while it is running on cruise control.

As waveform messages from sensory nerves combine with physiology feedback and enter the brain's mapping network through the limbic system, they can be observed by the self on the interference 'screens' of a particular cortex or a combination of cortices. (The self can also manipulate, prioritize and distort these incoming physiological waveforms through the amygdale, however.) As they blend in the cortex, the self is able to review the waveforms and if need be, respond with intention. By this time, however, the programming already in place to process the particular situation is also ready to respond.

Should a conscious 'executive' decision be made by the inner self, instructional waveforms are initiated through the prefrontal cortex. These are channeled through the motor cortex, which formats the waveforms for the hypothalamus. The hypothalamus in turn transduces these waveforms into physical response through the endocrine system and central nervous system. These instructional messengers may also contain a stop order to override whatever other instructions may already be in place.

Autonomic responses are established through initialized intentions and a subsequent programming of key web hubs by the mind. Most of these intentions are related to the survival of the body, translated from the self's fear of dying. This fear becomes translated into various scenarios that stimulate the programming features of mind. The programming waveforms stimulated by the mind are stored in neurons just as memories are, in the form of standing waves, crystallized by ionic molecular polarity and bonding sequences. Some autonomic programs are more permanently 'wired' into the standing waveforms that make up DNA bonds. These 'hard-wired' programs ultimately are passed on to the body's successors through the DNA.

These 'coded' standing waveforms with neurons are activated by certain types of waveforms incoming through sensory nerves and from interoception translated through the hypothalamus and thalamus. As information moves through this network, the neural programming indirectly relays the self's ultimate intentions of keeping the body alive with specific autonomic responses. The information will also be stepped up to the mind's web for viewing through the cortices. When we burn our finger, our autonomic programming will immediately respond by pulling the hand away. The self will also be able to view the incoming information separately, and initiate a separate, conscious response, such as tending to the injury or turning off the flame.

The inner self's recognition of information within the frontal cortex (or *mind screen*) is called *cognition*. In humans and primates, the central interface or bridge between the incoming impulse pathways of the nervous system and executive control is located in the *dorsolateral prefrontal cortex* (Otani 2002). It is here waveforms are examined, responded to and their responses relayed onto the motor cortex. Simultaneously, goal-directed intentions from the self stimulate the broadcast of waveform messages back into the neural net through the frontal cortex. Instructive waveforms are simultaneously pulsed through the hypothalamus, the specific regions of the motor cortex, and then broadcast throughout the nervous system.

These instructive waveforms together stimulate the various elemental channels to respond. In other words, the body is not shocked or jerked into motion solely from pulses moving out from the brain. There are several pathways of activity initiated during a full-body response. The body's endocrine systems are stimulated. The body's heat-producing centers are stimulated. The body's insulin and energy releasing centers are stimulated. The body's pacemaker, vasomotor, perfusive and respiratory functions all are simultaneously stimulated into immediate response. How else could the body react so instantaneously and thoroughly from head to toe following an intentional decision? We certainly have to characterize the chemical binding process as too cumbersome to exclusively provide these broadcasting mechanisms.

The connection between the cognitive functions of higher decision-making and the mind screen web are illustrated by the size of the frontal lobe cortex areas of the brain in more evolved organisms. Behavioral studies with animals and humans have also confirmed that complex executive functions with goal-directed behavior, language and higher cognition in general is associated with a larger, more developed prefrontal cortex (Fuster 2002). The developed frontal lobe cortex enables the self to command a greater volume of switchboard control and the ability to specify intention through a complex mental web. We also note that all highly evolved organisms have advanced backbones and high-energy entry-points to carry out full-body neural responses. As for less evolved organisms, we still find key neural regions that transduce conscious intentions, albeit with less complexly.

Microtubules

During the 1970s, Dr. Stewart Hameroff from the University of Arizona, and Dr. Kunio Yasue and Dr. Mari Jibu from the Okayama University began researching the pathways for conscious activity between neural cells. One of the mysteries they probed in independent research was how anesthesia agents such as chloroform and nitrous oxide could disable the consciousness of a patient. Through their respective research, they independently discovered that conscious activity within the body had to do with a curious matrix of twisted spiral filaments they called *tubulins.* These tubulins are arranged into networked pathways that wind through the neural cells in three-dimensional protein spirals called *microtubules.* These microtubules appear to be conducting tracts for waveform activity. The research illustrated that the microtubules make up a previously unseen network for subtle waveform biocommunication through the neural *dend-*

tritic web (Hameroff 1974; Hameroff 1982; Hameroff *et al.* 1984; Hameroff 1987; Hameroff and Penrose 1996, Hameroff 2010).

As the larger waveforms of the physical realm are processed and transmitted through dendrites, they conduct through the neurotransmitters between the synapses. As they are conducted through this medium, the waveforms meet with other waveforms traveling within the neural network. This convergence creates coherent interference patterns. The resonating results of these interference patterns are then transmitted through the subtle network of the microtubules. In this state, these subtle waveforms are 'stepped up' to a higher frequency format. These subtle high frequency waveforms in turn create holographic wave patterns, which are ultimately reflected (or mirrored) onto the 'screens' of the cortices. Once on the screens, these holograms interact with others to create a 'picture' of the physical body and the world around us. The inner self interacts with these cortices through the primary screening device of the frontal cortex to view this holographic picture.

Within these microtubules also travel the various subtle waveforms that conduct the intentions of the self through the body. The discovery of these microtubule pathways confirms much of the ancient wisdom of the *chakras, nadis* and *meridians*. These channels were also described as being pathways for living energy flow. We might consider nerve tracts as pathways of lower-frequency reflexive waveforms, while the microtubules broadcast higher-frequency, complex information waves.

We might compare the microtubular process of projecting wave interference patterns onto the mind to the recording of a musical composition in a modern studio. The studio producer will record the guitar onto one track, the piano onto another track, the drums onto another and the voice onto another track. The producer may even overlay background singers' voices onto other tracks. The producer will then assemble all the tracks together at particular sound levels to form the entire piece of music. This is often referred to as a *composition*. Each track makes up a piece of the total song. To listen to each track alone without the other tracks will sound weird. In much the same way, the mind captures the various waveform frequencies coming through the microtubular network, neural net and biochemical messengers — combining them to form unified images of the outside world.

This is the same principle as holography. One of the basic tenets of holography is that each part mirrors the entire image. This is accomplished through a splitting of waves as they interfere, creating a multitude of waves, each containing all the information via the composition of waveforms. Using waveform interference, the mind orchestrates holographic assembly in both directions. The mind reflects images semiconducted through particular neurons. The mind also stimulates effector neurons to act reflectively, using the pre-programming initiated by the intentions of the self.

The mindscreen projects combined images using the various cortex images — each from assembled waveforms from different locations. This collection of images is broadcast through crystallized neuron pathways. Each neuron is constructed with the appropriate crystal DNA structure, ion channel system and microtubules, giving it the ability to join with others to relay multiple waveform interference patterns simultaneously.

Memory

Modern neuroscience divides memory into short-term and long-term processes. Long-term memory is further divided into three types: *Episodic* — when memories are unique to the time and place; *semantic* — when memories involve concepts or learning; and *procedural* — when memories revolve around skills. Episodic memories relate to events that happened in the past, or people we knew from the past. Semantic memories relate more to concept understanding. Procedural memories relate to remembering how to ride a bike, write or use a telephone.

Interestingly, memory loss of one type will not typically accompany the loss of another type. Thus in many amnesia cases, long-term memory may appear erased while short-term memory is retained. The person may forget older events yet continue to remember what just happened.

Furthermore, all too frequently one type of long-term memory may be lost while another type is retained. For example, a person may suffer the loss of their episodic memory — forgetting their name, family, school history, phone number, birth date and other personal details. They might also forget events of the past. At the same time, they may remember how to write, drive, talk on the phone and even retain concepts such as how financial markets work.

Often a particular trauma or event may cause the forgetfulness of either what happened just before the event, or what happened just after the event. The former case is referred to as *retrograde amnesia* — a loss of memory just prior to a trauma. The latter is referred to as *anterograde amnesia* — a loss of memory just after a trauma. Both may also occur. The causes of these types of forgetfulness are considered quite mysterious. This is because memory has been miscalculated.

There are other types of memory loss. Many are unconnected to any particular event, while others follow injury to particular brain regions or involve trauma. Trauma-associated amnesia may or may not involve physical injury. It may follow a head injury or automobile accident. Traumatic amnesia may also follow the witnessing of a traumatic event, or may involve abuse. Rape is an example of traumatic amnesia involving abuse. *Psychogenic* or *dissociative fugue* is another type of memory loss, which also may occur following a trauma, and may result in a person identifying him- or herself as someone else, or even taking an unexpected trip to a place previously unknown. Other events that can cause memory loss include alcohol and drug related blackouts, and *Wernicke-Korsakoff's*, which is thought to be caused by thiamin deficiency.

A more common type of amnesia involves the loss of memory of a particular event. This may be the forgetting of certain childhood events, for example. Forgetting certain events may also be related to traumatic memory loss. Many of us forget events in the distant past that were not necessarily traumatic as well. It is not unusual for us to forget our younger childhood events. We also may recall something without remembering how we knew it—called *source amnesia.*

One illness overwhelming modern medicine and capturing research attention is *Alzheimer's disease.* The first documented case of AD was discovered by a Bavarian psychiatrist named Dr. Alois Alzheimer. Dr. Alzheimer treated a 51-year old patient who suffered from memory loss and hallucinations. The patient, "Auguste D" was frequently delirious and had extreme short-term memory deficit. She complained of having "lost myself." She was committed to the Frankfurt asylum in 1901 and died five years later. Autopsy revealed a sticky plaque among brain cells and nerve tissue entanglement. The disease was named after the diagnosis given by Dr. Alzheimer, and this variant of dementia became associated with physical damage to the brain apparently relating to a build-up of beta amyloid plaque among neurons.

The definite cause of AD has not been determined, although there appear to be a number of potential contributing factors. These include stress, free radical damage, heavy metal toxicity, and poor nutrition. Recent research seems to point at a lack of phosphatidylserine among brain cell membranes as well.

This sort of research contributes to our notion that memory is chemical-based. Meanwhile, EGG and magnetic resonance scans locate the seeming position for long-term memory storage location within the frontal and medial temporal lobes.

However, researchers have also found that—like motor function—memory storage has a high degree of plasticity. Research has disclosed numerous instances where memories are moved to different regions of the brain. This has especially been found in situations of stroke or other brain damage.

The plasticity of memory is also evident following hemicortication surgeries—a frequent treatment of childhood epilepsy for many years. Episodic memories were retained even through the brain regions known to retain episodic memories were removed. We must therefore question the assumption that memories are specific to particular neurons.

Yet we still need to address the fact that many memory losses occur following brain damage. So are memories physical or not?

The first clue is that most of these cases are specific to short-term memory loss. Long-term memories remain a mystery. In one study (Piolino *et al.* 2006), thirteen patients with early stage dementia, ten patients with semantic dementia and fifteen patients with frontotemporal dementia were compared to assess the connection between memory loss and damage to the medial temporal lobe. One of the central areas of focus in this study was the *autobiographical amnesia of episodic memories,* or the lack of ability to acquire or remember past events.

The results of this study concluded no consistency between memory loss and frontal lobe impairment. In some cases, short-term memories were difficult to acquire as a whole, and in other cases, the memory acquisition depended upon the details and importance of the event. In many cases, long-term "remote" memories were retained and preserved, while short-term details and events were not. This led the study authors to support a newer theory called the *multiple trace theory,* which says that memory acquisition occurs through more than one physical mechanism, and can be stored in multiple locations in the brain.

In a similar study (Matuszewski *et al.* 2006) on autobiographical episodic memory loss among frontotemporal dementia patients, near learning abilities with semantic memories revealed a shifting executive function with multiple processes. As for other possible models of memory acquisition, several studies have indicated that the hippocampus complex was significantly involved in the storage and recall of recent memories, but not for older memories. Other research has offered evidence that the hippocampus complex is responsible for autobiographical episodic memory and special memory, but the storage of other types of memory was shifted to other locations (Nadel and Moscovitch 1997).

In a 2002 report (Nester *et al.*) published in *Neuropsychologia* on autobiographical memories among semantic dementia patients, the preservation of recent memories and the loss of remote memories supported the trace theory of memory retention and acquisition. This report confirms, as so many cruel animal studies have, that memories are not chemically retained within specific neurons.

Thus, we can logically compare memories to data stored on a computer's hard drive. Modern science has yet to fathom the processes that must fall in place to stack, sort and assemble memory information into electromagnetic neuron storage locations, however.

This stems primarily from the fact that modern science does not understand the most basic fundamental of biology: the *driver* of the living organism. We must understand the source of operation first. Then we can functionally understand the organism's operation. Just as a car needs a driver to operate. Once we realize the role of the driver of the car, we can see how the driver uses the wheel, the clutch and the gas pedal to move the car.

The driver of the body utilizes particular equipment to drive the body. The brain is like the instrument panel, and the mind is like the software driving the instrument panel. Like the driver of the car, the inner self dictates the functioning of the body. Rather than an instrument panel, steering wheel, gas pedal and brake system, the self uses the mind, the prefrontal cortex, motor cortex and limbic system to execute commands to the body.

This was exposed in a study of memory-challenged patients with different brain disorders (Thomas-Anterion 2000). Twelve Alzheimer's disease patients and twelve frontotemporal dementia patients with functionally similar semantic memory, logical memory and retrograde memory test scores were studied for antegrade verbal memory and frontal lobe activity. Despite similar memory acquisition scores and types of memory loss, physiological brain function occurred in different locations among the subjects. This illustrated flexibility in brain region utilization, quite similar to practical daily living: Should we be unable to pick up something with one hand, we will quickly adjust and pick up the item with the other hand. In the same way, the self, using the utility of the mind, can often accomplish the same purpose using different neurons, cortices and/or limbic components.

This doesn't contradict the notion that should the brain's neurons be struck with a debilitating disease or injury, the inner self may not be able to utilize the instruments of the brain to recall and retain memories. Memory is in fact a handshaking process between the mind's programming, the sensory system, the hippocampus complex, the various cortices, and the inner self.

Indeed, memory can be retained using a variety of physical mechanisms. Humans have utilized various physical tools besides brain cells to replace or augment memory function for thousands of years. A person may retain memories using a diary to assist in the recall of particular thoughts, emotions and events. Projects or objectives may be recorded onto daily planners, electronic smart phones, or digital voice recorders for later recall. Most students and businesspeople carry notebooks to every class or meeting to assist with the retention and recall of lectures and discussions. These external memory devices replace or augment limited memorization functions. They also illustrate the inner self's intention to remember.

The memory experiments by Dr. Wilder Penfield at the Montreal Neurological Institute in the 1970s clearly illustrated that memories typically accompanied emotions and intentions. When Dr. Penfield's weak electrical currents excited locations within the brain, the subject would recall historical facts associated with past experiences. Their recollections included songs connected to feelings from the past, aromas connected to experiences, people connected to personal relationships, and events connected to other emotional events. Dry information such as what score a person received twenty years ago on a test or sporting event might seem like raw data, but this data can be connected to personal intentions to win or receive a good score. Without an emotional, intentional attachment, the ability to recall that event subsides as the self's intention to remember it weakens.

What this tells us is that memory is impossible without emotional intention or consciousness. Memory studies have shown that when a person is emotionally involved in a particular incident or detail, the recall rate of that incident or detail is significantly higher. Furthermore, as the event converts to longer-term memory, if it has no emotional attachment, it is typically sorted out during our consolidation process — which typically takes place as we sleep. In order to remember trivial details, those subjects who connect the detail to a colorful, emotional or funny association will dramatically increase the likelihood of recalling it later.

Without consciousness there would be no need for memory or recall. We might think that a robot must have a memory in order to store its programming information. However, no robot would be built without the original intention produced by consciousness. Without consciousness, there would be no purpose for a robot. The robot, then, is simply a surrogate of a conscious person's purpose and intention. This is precisely what the physical body is.

We can logically conclude that the inner self utilizes the physical elements of the brain for memory retention and recall, but only by utilizing the programming of the mind. This also means that damage to the brain's hardware may also destroy the organism's ability to mentally recall and apply those memories. Memorization and recall may be shifted to a variety of brain regions and even external tools. Some hardware is still necessary, however. This is because physical information is perceived through interference patterns of electromagnetic waveforms. These interference patterns become crystallized within groups of resonating neurons.

This information will not be retrievable without conscious intention. Should those brain cells become damaged, those memories may become difficult to retrieve, but not impossible. The self could still retrieve them through investigating other physical evidence such as a photo album.

Memory retrieval is interrupted by broken links between the inner self and those interference patterns. The standing waveforms may still be crystallized within the neurons. Or the neurons may be damaged. Then they will not be able to retain the crystallized waveform patterns. These two possibilities are also associated: A broken link can precipitate from unused neurons and damage to the neurons.

We can compare memory and neurons to wind and sailboat sails. If the sail rips, the boat will not be able to ride the wind. The wind may be blowing, but since the sail is ripped, the sail cannot catch the wind and drive the boat.

As to whether the forgetfulness associated with dementia or Alzheimer's disease indicates that the inner self chooses to forget: This can be a cruel supposition to those family and friends surrounding the dementia patient. Certainly the dementia patient may not have chosen specifically to forget their family and friends. At the same time, we must recognize that there are deeper issues involved. The inner self may be dealing with a deep desire to escape the trivial requirements and responsibilities brought on by their family and friends. This may be something they have not dealt with directly in their life. They may not have drawn the appropriate boundaries, and/or have shouldered more than they are comfortable with. So the physical consequence that resolves the need to draw boundaries is to shut off those connections and responsibilities.

There may also be a natural desire to be finished with the pettiness of this world. The inner self may be withdrawing gradually as a matter of natural course. They may have been subjected to the life-saving therapies of modern care, and their physical body may well be outliving the inner self's natural time of death. This "internal clock" of time within the body is upset by modern technology.

For example, a stroke has the potential to shut off circulation to the brain. Under natural conditions, this would be fatal. In a modern hospital trauma center, however, physicians can often clear the blockage of the blood vessel to the brain with stents, micro-balloons and other methods. The result is an extension of the person's life beyond the naturally-appointed time of death.

The natural result of a stroke leads to the potential for brain cells to undergo damage due to their having a lack of blood flow. Ordinarily, this should cause death.

The continued survival of the body as a result of the trauma center's efforts may also lead to a loss of brain activity. Instead of naturally resulting in death, the inner self is stuck inside a body with damaged brain cells.

The inner self may also respond to a personal trauma that has shocked the self into withdrawing. This may be related to the loss of a spouse or another loved one's physical body. This may prompt the inner self to question why the other person left them behind. Why are they being left alone? This emotional trauma, perhaps combined with brain neuron damage, can easily lead to the withdrawal of the inner self from family members and certain types of memories.

In Alzheimer's disease, for example, many researchers have pointed to free radical damage to polyunsaturated fatty acids that surround brain cells. With this increased oxidative damage comes the mysterious formation of amyloid-beta plaque within the neurons. The conventional understanding was that these Abeta fibrils were the predictive element of AD.

New evidence indicates that Abeta oligomers circulating amongst neurons and cerebrospinal fluid take place before neuron damage. One study found that greater Abeta oligomers circulating within the cerebrospinal fluid was a precursor for later AD (Fukumoto *et al.* 2010).

These problems are compounded by circulatory deficiencies: Reduced nutrient supply due to narrowed arteries caused by oxidative LDL and other radical species.

The progressive release of oligomers and the assembly of neurotoxic amyloid fibrils or plaques appear to arise from an enzyme called acetylcholinesterase.(Walsh *et al.* 2007) So now the question becomes, what stimulates the release of this enzyme?

Enzymes are complicated structures. They are proteins that are produced by the RNA and/or ribosomes within the cells. A specialized enzyme such as acetylcholinesterase is stimulated and put into action through a complex process related to the epigenetic system we discussed earlier. As we discussed, the epigenetic system responds to a mixture of environmental stimuli and the inner self's response to that stimuli. This response in turn triggers epigenetic marks on the DNA, which turn on genes that process certain functions.

What this all means is that the mechanism of Abeta plaque and subsequent damage to brain cells is ultimately linked to the condition of the inner self. The inner self, in response to environment, emotional state or outlook in general, indirectly stimulates the process of Abeta oligomer production—ultimately stimulating the eventual progression of amyloid-beta plaque around the nerve cells.

This indicates the radical possibility that Alzheimer's and dementia are ultimately rooted within the inner self. The role of the inner self as the driver of the mental and physical mechanisms of memory is not simply incidental: it is causal.

The relationship between visual pictures, imagination and memory are linked to the context of the inner self as the intentional viewer. The inner self programs the mind's reflective imagery. The holographic pictures reflected onto the mindscreen are constructed by a combination of retinal cells, the optic nerve, the LGM, neurons from the visual cortex, together with the intentions of the inner self. We might refer to this process as *focus.* Through conscious intent, the self can also stimulate the mind to construct pictures using only previously-captured and internalized images. We can aptly refer to this as *imagination.* Through a combination of focus and imagination, intentional pictures are constructed within the mind.

When attached to an intentional picture or image, incoming information can be sorted and stored onto to the neural net. When we connect information with images—including any sensual input such as sound or touch—we are effectively multiplying the number of references within that data. We might compare this with how search engine spiders prioritize web pages. The spiders will travel the net and count the cross referencing of websites to determine a ranking of popularity between websites. In the same way, the mind's programming prioritizes images by the number of links to the interests of the inner self. In other words, the self instructs the mind to prioritize memories by interest: The more intentional screenings each image has, the higher its priority ranking. The higher its priority ranking, the more available the mind makes that memory.

As a result, our retrievable memories of the past are usually connected to experiences that affected the inner self somehow. This means they had emotional effects upon the inner self. Once the self has attached an emotional experience to an image, the sense perception or image is indelibly attached to that emotion. These attached sense perceptions have now become *impressions.* By attaching the inner self's objectives (emotions) to sounds, smells, touch, or visual images, we are effectively cataloging the perception with the prioritization of that emotion. The more important the emotion, the higher the perception ranks in memory.

An example of this emotional attachment is how a song will reconnect us back to a precise time and place of our chronological past. Because the original hearing of the song became attached to the emotions of the inner self, the hearing of the song later will stimulate the recall of vivid memories of those times. These may include details otherwise long forgotten.

This can work with pictures just as well. We may see a particular picture and be reminded of the time, place and details surrounding the moment when that picture was taken. The images in the picture stimulated the retrieval of the emotions just as the song did in the previous example.

Why does the memory work better when connected to emotional attachments? What is it about a picture, song, or funny story from our past that enables us to retrieve vivid memories?

Remember that information travels through the neural network through varying waveforms that interact to become combined images or information. This combination could be compared to throwing several stones into a small pond. Each ripple created by a stone is connected to the weight and size of the stone itself. As the different ripples from the different stones collide, they create an interaction of multiple waves. This interaction of ripples creates a rich multi-layered view of the history of the stone throws. An observer of the interactive rippling could assess a total picture of what kinds of stones were dropped into the pond.

This is analogous to how a television screen converts various colors, forms, and sounds onto the viewing screen to image an original broadcast. As various radio wave signals are received by the antenna or cable input, they are flashed interactively upon the screen. It is this interaction that creates the whole picture. The individual radio waves by themselves would not communicate much. It is their interactivity with the polarity of the screen that renders them understandable.

In other words, outside the physical brain's issues and the back-and-forth process of checking and crosschecking between the mind and the neural network lies the conscious intent of the self. The self drives the process of the mind's information processing software. The self also ultimately drives the *extent* of the memory saved and retrieved.

While we can typically remember many interesting things about our life and retrieve them quite easily without much effort, we have to make a conscious effort to remember details that are less important to us. If we want to remember details taught in a science class for example, we have to make a concerted effort to repeatedly focus on the information in order to retain them and repeat them later. Simply listening to the lecture and hearing the information once typically does not allow the attachment and recall of massive amounts of unimportant details onto the mind's memory web. We might want good grades, but we may not be interested in the information itself. We do not have any emotional attachment to it. We will have to listen to it, read about it, write it down and then maybe read about it again in hopes that we will somehow connect enough emotion to the information to remember it. If we are able to utilize some of the methods mentioned above—relating the details to unique pictures and funny stories—our ability to remember these details will be better. The remembrance is occurring because the self is connecting emotional intention to the information.

For this same reason, we tend to better remember details about the things that interest us the most. For example, we often see men and boys able to remember the batting averages of their favorite baseball players. Yet they are unable to remember the latest economic statistics—even though they saw both on the same television news show. Here the details of intended hobbies and personal missions are placed in a higher priority. We have focused greater intention upon the details we remembered.

This is illustrated by a study published in 2005 (Lindstrom *et al.*) concluding that a positive relationship existed between acquiring later-in-life Alzheimer's disease and increased television viewing among middle-aged adults. 135 elderly Alzheimer's cases and 331 healthy (control) subjects were interviewed and classified for television viewing duration during their mid-life years. The results found that for each hour per day of mid-life television viewing, Alzheimer's occurrence increased 1.3 times. Conversely, intellectually stimulating activities and social activities were associated with lower Alzheimer's rates. The study's authors concluded that social engagement with others somehow better utilized the neurons at risk of dementia-related disorders.

While watching television, the self's focus becomes increasingly tied to the virtual illusions of the tele-scripted drama, as opposed to the variegated living world around us. These adults presumably reach for their escape from the world by watching television because they prefer to *unfocus* their attention on the living world. (This assumes fictional dramas—not news and documentary programs reflecting reality.) Perhaps the living world provides too many problems or difficulties to solve. Conversely, social activities engage the self's attention onto the real lives and problems of the world. This requires further emotional involvement from the self. Life requires us to prioritize the mass of incoming information. This stresses the neural mechanisms—keeping them better exercised.

The real world also stimulates the self to utilize the tools of the mind to solve the problems of the physical world. Many studies have confirmed that mental exercises and problem solving create better cognition and a more resilient memory.

In the case of television watchers, the self's lack of focus and work on real world problems leads to a slow degeneration of biocommunication pathways. Like unused muscles, the neurons are under-utilized. They receive less circulation, less detoxification, less interaction and less activity. This all leads to the slow degeneration of those cells, opening them up to accumulating ameloid beta plaque or a myriad of brain-stifling developments.

In the final analysis, it is the propensity of the inner self to escape from reality that under-utilizes the brain's biocommunication equipment. Does this mean the self wills or intends the Alzheimer's scenario? Not directly, but just as a sedentary lifestyle perpetuates obesity and an inability to adequately move and exercise, the propensity to escape certain physical realities perpetuates a progressive inability to utilize certain regions of the brain.

It has long been held by sleep researchers — who have measured the brain's electrical activity during sleep — that the higher electrical activity from individual brain neurons indicates that during sleep the neurons are reassembling and sorting information received during the day. The neurons are processing this information into long-term memory. This is referred to as *consolidation*. This theory has recently been challenged by memory researchers who have noticed that the limbic system and interference processes appear to be the focal point of the higher electrical activity. As Dr. John Wixted, professor of Psychology at the University of California at San Diego proposed in 2005, the evidence seems to point to interference mechanics created by waking and sleeping activities. The process of sleep apparently provokes priorities or images that interfere with the consolidation process of memories.

We would contend this is caused by those initial memories not being highly prioritized by the intentions of the self. For this reason, not all the recent memory is eliminated during sleep. The memories considered more critical to the self are retained. Otherwise, how could we remember those things we consider dear (beyond a day) and forget the other details?

Where do the memory waveform interference patterns go as our intentions distance them? Where do the waveforms not imaged by the mind go? Do they still exist somewhere?

The conscious mind is a mapping and screening mechanism driven by the self. It is conscious because it is driven by consciousness. The self, however, is of another nature: The self is *composed of* consciousness. Waveform interference patterns continue to exist in the larger realm of consciousness. However, the bridle of misidentification confines the self to those interference patterns intentionally collected and translated by the limbic system, and projected by the mind. The brain and mind are simply tools for intention. This might be comparable to a person going to a lecture and choosing to write down notes on the lecture, even though the person could certainly just listen to the lecture and remember the interesting parts of the lecture. The uninteresting data will likely remain outside the memory web because the self is not interested in it. The notes, on the other hand, will be available to the self because of the intentions of the self to pass the class.

This also means that the mind mechanism is limited by and focused onto the intentions of the self. Therefore, the mind will sometimes alter or ignore inputs that do not fit with the intentions of the self. As a result, the self will not want to maintain a memory that might conflict with its attempts to enjoy the physical world. Most traumas are erased from the "conscious" awareness of the mind simply because the self does not want to face those painful experiences. However, if the inner self does not learn and grow from the experience, the self cannot release its focus upon the trauma. As a result, the waveform interference patterns of the trauma event continue to be linked to the emotions of the self—which forces the memory to be retained and linked to those emotions. Linked with these emotions, the memory is prioritized near the top of the standing wave hierarchy, forcing the self to continue to see the images of that memory until it is resolved.

Again, it is only when the trauma has been resolved by the self that the emotion can be removed from the memory. When the emotional link is removed from the memory, it becomes a worthless detail to the self, and the mind eventually consolidates it and deprioritizes it. Over time, this reprioritization routine of the mind's programming releases the details, and the memory is gradually downgraded within the memory net.

The question becomes; how does the self resolve the trauma? This is accomplished through growth and learning. The self must determine why the event happened. The self must forgive the person who we might be holding responsible. The self must come to an understanding regarding the event and the people involved. The self must learn from the event what was supposed to be learned. As soon as this takes place, the self can detach from the event and move on. This is often communicated by the expression: *"What do I need to learn from this experience?"* If we do not know, we will probably continue to hold onto it.

Reprioritization or consolidation does not eliminate the event. It still exists in waveform interference pattern form. However, ones mental memory of an event is inseparable from intent. As long as there is intent to remember it—or an emotion connected to it—the waveform will be accessible. This might be compared again to the internet. While so many websites might be out there—some even communicating hatred or violence—we choose to only surf the websites we are interested in. We will ignore those others, and even though they may still be there and possibly even accessible, the web surfer will probably not even be aware of their existence.

On the other hand, should we not learn and grow from a trauma, we may instead seek to escape from it. This can lead to drug and alcohol abuse, and other strategies of escape. It can also lead to the slow progression of dementia.

It is apparent that the self has the ability to be selective in terms of memory. The self has the ability to choose its viewing priorities. Reflecting this, the limbic system's memory sorting facilities can also be directed with selectivity. This is why we remember interesting things more than boring things. This is also why we can forget traumatic events during childhood while remembering all too clearly the traumatic events that unfolded during adolescence or adulthood. During times of childhood trauma, the inner self can more easily disconnect from the event. This ease of disconnection helps the memory fade. A trauma occurring later in life will have a lot more emotional attachment than a trauma occurring during youth. For this reason, it is clinically more difficult to resolve traumas that occur after 5-7 years of age.

We might also consider how children can run around laughing and playing, and when they fall—especially if they are playing a game they enjoy—they may simply jump up and keep playing. They may hardly notice the scrapes and scratches—or the pain—of the trauma. The child may even avoid Mom's first aid application—intended to avoid infection and speed healing. In the child's eyes, this might just interfere with the remainder of the game.

It is likely this child will completely forget this trauma as he or she quickly learns not to repeat the fall. Should an adult have such a fall there would likely be significantly more trauma. An adult will likely become embarrassed for such a fall. This would be combined with an increased focus on the ramifications of the fall: Will it get infected? Will the knee be injured for long? Will the fall cause any major disabilities? As the adult's mind plays out all the emotional fears of the self within, the fall soon becomes embedded into long(er) term memory storage.

This type of focus also contributes to our ability to remember one person's name while forgetting another's. It is not that the person whose name we forgot did not interest us: Their name simply did not capture our emotional focus at the moment. Our mind was engaged in processing other items that took priority over the name. The mind is the programming tool of the inner self, and though it might seem a bit out of control at times, its sub-routines directly or indirectly respond to the interests of the self. Should we exert a determined effort to remember names, however, it would be another story. We would likely employ various *mnemonic* tools such as creating a funny picture to associate with the person's name. These intentional insertions are stimulated by the self, but are executed through the amygdala.

Once the mind creates that funny picture, it is inserted by the amygdala into the limbic system, which exchanges a holographic image with the frontal cortex. The self thus becomes emotionally involved directly in the process of viewing a holographic representation of the name via this mechanism. This intentional viewing triggers a priority sort of the memory within the hippocampus — enabling better retention and recall of the name.

The processes of the mind work through a combination of programming, design, and the intentional steering by the self. The self may drive or direct the mind, but does not necessarily control the design of the mechanism. There are some benefits of this. Imagine a situation where a person remembered every trauma experienced during their lifetime: The pain of being enclosed in the womb; the trauma of being born; the challenges of growing up; the pain of every accident or physical injury. Each of these events is certainly traumatic. If we were to remember every one vividly, we would be tormented to say the least. The reason why we do not remember these earlier traumas is because we quickly learned the lessons they presented to us.

The interaction between the self and the amygdala — the emotional center of the limbic system — and the memory-oriented regions of the limbic system such as hippocampus, hypothalamus and the visual cortex, have been shown in EEG and magnetic resonance studies. The prefrontal cortex — often referred to as the *seat of cognitive control* — is able to modulate these waveform interactions. This modulation provides the ability to interfere in the memory stacking and prioritization processes, thereby producing memory suppression or repression.

In research performed in the Department of Psychology at the University of Colorado (Depue *et al.* 2006), subjects were shown faces paired with either pictures or other faces — some neutral and some disturbing. After repetition and memorization, the subjects underwent brain MRIs while being asked to either recall an image paired with a particular face, or suppress the image. This gave researchers the ability to trace the regions of the brain involved with both memory recall and suppression. The study concluded firstly that people are able to successfully suppress disturbing images upon request. This is a substantial point. In addition, MRI scans demonstrated the involvement of the prefrontal cortex in memory suppression. The inner self has a considerable amount of control over our memories, using the prefrontal cortex to exercise this control.

This relationship between memory and intention has been taught for many decades by a number of memory experts. Some have written and lectured on a process of using emotion to build *super-memories*. There also have been many demonstrations by those who have utilized these methods and developed super-memories. The basic technique is to connect the detail to be re-membered to an interesting image and/or story. This creates an emotional connection with the detail. A number of details can thus be memorized by linking them together into a series of im-ages to create a funny or unique story.

Forgetting is not necessarily a bad thing, however. An exam-ple to consider is Solomon Shereshevskii (1886-1958), a Russian journalist who seemed to remember just about everything. Solomon could remember extensive lists of numbers, facts, de-tails, names and faces. He was truly one of history's greatest memorizers. His method of remembering such detail, it was later discovered, was due to his ability to connect each fact or figure to a three-dimensional visual picture. Doing this would allow him to relate each fact to not only a particular visual picture, but one that had personal character. This inserted emotion into the memory sorting process.

Over time, Solomon had problems with his super-memory. He would not recognize acquaintances years after meeting them because their faces had aged—he had remembered their earlier faces too clearly, it seemed. He was also tormented with the vast amount of details he retained. As a result, Solomon spent his later years lost in daydreams and reveries, as his bank of vivid memories crowded out new experiences.

Subconsciousness

The theories and concepts proposed by Dr. Janet and Dr. Freud not much more than a century ago included the notion of the subconscious mind. Hypnosis provided the basis for these conclusions. Under hypnosis, patients demonstrated an awareness of events and information seemingly unavailable to their conscious minds during their normal awakened states.

Because our 'conscious' minds appear not to be aware of the subtle memory programming mechanisms of the mind, the concept of a subconscious mind appeared to adequately explain these phenomena. We must question this assumption, however. What is this mysterious subconsciousness? Why can a person who is brought under trance—which is simply a state of suggestion and trust—suddenly be able to recall things that are not otherwise recalled? How does the programming of the mind otherwise operate beneath the awareness of the conscious mind? Furthermore, what is dreaming?

The empirical understanding of the existence of a transcendental inner self seamlessly explains these mysteries. It is precisely the positioning of the inner self—the operator—within the body that creates the ability of the mind to submit to the suggestion of hypnosis. The self simply makes a determination to submit to suggestion, and the body and mind follow.

It is the cloaking of the self by the veil of misidentification that is responsible for the mysterious nature of the inner self. Yet it is the permanence of the inner self throughout the changing physical body that allows the recall of unmemorized events under hypnosis. This is because, after all, the self still experienced these events, even though their mental links are gone.

Although the mind and its programming are set up based upon the intentions of the self, the mind is still different from the self. The mind has its own design, and sometimes the mind can get out of control of the self. As the mind's programming is developed, it can take us to places we ultimately do not want to go. It can be carried away with the directives we have given it. The main directive the self gives the mind is to figure out ways to achieve physical pleasure. The mind begins to concoct various scenarios for physical enjoyment. Sometimes these scenarios will cross the line of decency or morality. The self is clearly aware of these lines. However, the mind will also produce—should the self be open to them—various justifications for the activity to appeal to the morality of the self. We will then be faced with a moral decision on whether to do something or not. As this decision is being made, the mind will continue to throw justifications for the activity on the screen for the self to review.

This is how we evolve and grow as individuals. As the mind presents us with choices, we have the ability to make decisions. These decisions can utilize the resource of intelligence. Through intelligence, we can decide to move the body in such a way that causes the least amount of frustration and pain upon others. Or we can decide to seek our own pleasure first and foremost.

Many times nature designs consequences that force a choice between our own pleasure and our relationships. This forces us to consider whether our own pleasure is more important to us than our relationships with others. This conflict between the self's desire for pleasure and the desire to unselfishly love is an oft-repeating lesson for each of us.

In a beautiful symphony of homunculus reflection, humans have invented and assembled televisions, computers and programs to almost precisely reflect the functionality of our brains and mental programming. This adds to the confirmation that our mental and physical programming stems from an intention self. Like our minds and brains, computers and televisions are simply reflections of the desires and objectives of a conscious inner self.

Without the driving force of an intentional self there would be no need for information. We cannot train a dead rat to do tricks. Neither can we expect a dead man to remember names by shouting those names into the body's ears.

All the brain regions and brain cells will still be intact in a newly deceased dead body. Yet there is no mind running the brain because there is no intention. The transcendental self has left the body. The electromagnetic waveform pulses of the brain stop, and the mind slowly dissolves.

Mental Death

This is not to say the inner self has no memory without the brain. This is clearly evidenced by near death experiences and past life regression research. The inner self has the ability to recall events regardless of whether they entered the frontal cortex through the sensory system. In clinical death experiences, the body may lie brain-dead on the hospital bed, yet the self will remember the experience and even recalls many events occurring around the hospital bed and among relatives that could not otherwise be seen.

During this point of clinical death—as we'll discuss further in the next chapter—the eyes are closed and brain activity has stopped. Why is there factual observation and memory without a functioning brain and sensory system?

Consistent with the religious teachings of the Hebrews, Moslems, Christians, Hindus, Taoists, Buddhists and so many other religious faiths, and consistent with the philosophies of the Greeks, Egyptians, Mayans, Aborigines, Polynesians, North American Indians and other ancient societies, the inner self has a spiritual identity—transcendental to this physical dimension. This identity has been described variously as spirit, soul or angel, while its home has been called the spiritual world, heaven and the transcendental world.

This spiritual being has the ability to retain and remember everything in the past and present, assuming the self is not currently locked up within the confines of the false identification of the physical body and mind.

Just as a dark movie theater blocks our ability to see what is going on around us as we focus upon a movie, our absorption into our current mental concoctions and present physical body buries the self with a mountain of illusion. In a movie theater, it is dark and the screen in front of us is very large. This set up makes us focus on the movie. We temporarily escape our real lives as we focus on the drama of the movie. While we do not necessarily forget the outside world exists (as we do while we are within a physical body) we can become involved in the movie to the point where we empathize with the movie's characters and become entranced by the plot. While we are entranced by the plot and characters, we are not focused on our own lives. Momentarily, we forget our own lives as we focus on the movie.

This is a similar state we are in now, except that our focus is more complete. The "movie" the mind and physical world presents to us is so real and involving, that we soon forget our real identities. We can see this among children, as their childlike approach to the world becomes replaced with the practical realities of the world. *The true nature of the self is, in fact, very childlike.*

Going back to the movie analogy; we can also get a perspective of the mind's death. When we are watching the movie's plot unfold, we become focused on the various details of the movie. If it is a mystery, we are focused upon the details of each character with respect to whether they could have committed the crime. Once the movie is over and we leave the theater, this "movie plot focus" fades away. Once the projector has stopped, we are no longer concerned about the nuances of each character. We now see the movie for what it was: a dramatic illusion meant to entertain us. As we walk out of the movie, we consider the movie's overall qualities: What did we learn from it? Was the plot consistent? Did we like the ending? This overreaching perspective on the movie is similar to the self's inner perspective upon the physical world.

While we are in the body, we are focused upon the practical realities of the world. We become involved in each character, and each event becomes dramatic and consequential. Our mind gets wound up among these events as it records all the details and plays back all the feedback/response loops.

Our current mind might be compared to looking at a pond after many stones have been tossed into it. The confluence of its intersecting and interfering ripples contain the information the observer is focused upon. Those interference patterns reveal the immediate history of how many stones were thrown in and how they thrown in.

However, once the self leaves the body, the electricity within the body stops. There is no nervous activity to stimulate electromagnetic waves. There is no stimulation of our central nervous system to gain sensory feedback or biochemical reception. These functions all stop as the self is released from the gross physical body.

When this activity stops, the mind also dissolves. The mind simply evaporates, just as a pond becomes still when there is no wind, no current, and nothing thrown into it. The gross mind dies when the body dies.

This does not mean that the consciousness of the self does not continue. The desires, goals, objectives and direction of the self continue to exist. These move with the self much like an aroma moves with a person's body. Just as the person who just left the movie carries with him the experience created by the movie's ending, the self carries away the overall effects of the physical lifetime. These include the sum effects of our activities upon others, the desires we bring away and the relationships we have made.

Mind Games

Again, the inner self is separate from the mind. The inner self is the user of the mind's programming, and the viewer of the mindscreen. By understanding how the mind's programming bridges the self with the physical body, we can better understand how we perceive the world. We can understand how we incorrectly identify ourselves as physical bodies, and we can understand how we misjudge the temporary the physical world as permanent.

The goals and intentions of the inner self are converted to practical strategies by the mind. The mind is a subtle programming tool that embraces the intentions of the inner self, and designs processes to most effectively execute those intentions. Because the mind operates within the construct of waveform mechanics, it is designed to manipulate and coordinate waveforms through and between the senses and nervous system. Utilizing this ability gives the mind the opportunity to sort and arrange the waveforms that accomplish its programming goals. It prioritizes the various wave patterns moving through the body, and assembles various concoctions based on the data it receives.

The mind is very impressionable and adaptable. From conception, the mind begins to utilize the incoming wave patterns from the senses to sort through the nature of the body's environment. It also utilizes the various feedback impulses from within the body to coordinate physiological nerve centers.

The similarity between the mind's mechanisms and artificial intelligence software is uncanny. Artificial intelligence may seem to be running on automatic, but its programs were designed by conscious programmers. The mind is also programmed by a conscious programmer. The AI programmer writes software code with plenty of "IF" and "THEN" statements to create learning loops. Just as in artificial intelligence, the mind's programming also responds to its inputs and outputs and learns new methods to adapt to external parameters.

The self has two prime directives for the mind. These are love and pleasure. The self yearns for love and pleasure, and our fulfillment is based upon accomplishing these. Based on these two primary commands from the self, the mind develops various strategies to manipulate the body and the environment to accomplish these realities. If one strategy is unsuccessful in fulfilling the self's ultimate goals, the mind will then develop yet another strategy. These are called *concoctions.* They are the mind's recipes for accomplishing the goals of the self.

These mental strategies or concoctions developed by the mind are frequently reviewed by the inner self. As a result, the self becomes deeply involved and even committed to the concoctions of the mind. This is because achieving love and pleasure through the physical world using a physical body is not an easy accomplishment. As the self becomes committed to the mind's strategies, determination develops. As the self becomes determined, the self will rest its hopes of accomplishing its primary directives by achieving the mind's current strategic concoctions.

A good example illustrating this is how our primary directive for obtaining true love evolves with the mind's various strategies. In the beginning of life within a particular body, the self attempts to receive true love from the body's parents. After a few years of trying to please the body's parents without achieving the satisfaction of true love, the inner self feeds back to the mind that parental love is not achieving the primary directive.

As a result, the mind concocts—after observing others playing and laughing with their friends—that achieving certain relationships with others should complete the directive. During youth, friendships with playmates may subsequently become the goal.

Once these relationships still do not satisfy the primary directive of the inner self, achieving a relationship with the opposite sex may become the current concoction of the mind. The mind develops various strategies to accomplish this, such as becoming successful in sports, school, popularity, and so on—all to gain admiration.

Once a girlfriend/boyfriend relationship is achieved, after some time again the self will still not be satisfied. The primary directive of pure love has not been reached. The mind may then contrive that maybe marriage will accomplish the goal. *Maybe if we possessed the other person,* the mind proposes. We soon discover that this possession was an illusion, and not fulfilling to boot. Disappointed, the self then directs the mind to look elsewhere for the attention and admiration of others in its attempt to gain the love the self needs.

To accomplish this, the mind develops strategies such as becoming successful in a particular career or skill. This strategy is based upon the observation that others who have become successful have achieved the admiration of others. The mind concludes that if we can be seen as a success, we will achieve others' love—again a failed assumption, as the many suicides by famous people have shown us.

As the self feeds back to the mind that we still have not accomplished the fulfillment we need, the mind will develop yet another strategy. On this process goes. The mind keeps concocting new strategies. Once one fails, another is concocted to replace it.

This same process works for the other primary directive: pleasure. The self is constantly looking for pleasure, and this is fed into the mind to try to achieve pleasure in the physical world. The mind concocts various strategies to achieve pleasure. During the early years, this may consist of getting certain toys and games. Later on, the concoctions will become more complex, including obtaining wealth, a new house, or perhaps a new location that appears to the mind to be more beautiful or warmer than the body's current location.

These larger concoctions are filled in with more immediate concoctions such as eating a tasty meal, having sex, watching a movie or television, or listening to a particular song or concert. These strategies large and small are developed by the mind, and because the self wants to achieve the directive, the body is engaged to accomplish those strategies. With each successive failure, the mind immediately comes up with yet another new strategy.

The process may not be as orderly as laid out above, however. The mind will concoct numerous strategies concurrent to the body's execution of any one. At any one time, the body may be executing several strategies the mind may have concocted.

Each strategy of the mind assumes success. Hence, the self anticipates that once a particular concoction of the mind is accomplished, the goal will be met. As we can observe in our lives and in the lives of others, the mind's concoctions never seem to satisfy either of the two central intentions of the self for achieving love and pleasure. The problem lies with a non-physical, transcendental person looking for fulfillment within a physical realm.

This does not mean that the mind is in charge of the self, however. The inner self has the ultimate jurisdiction over the mind. The self has veto power. The self approves the mind's general concoctions before the body can engage. Much of the time, this veto power is not well used, however. Most of us will just follow whatever the mind concocts, with little argument. The self incorrectly assumes that the mind must be on to something.

Why is this assumption not correct? Just consider: How many of us are actually fulfilled by following the mind's concoctions? In fact, those of us who simply follow the mind's concoctions without question are quite miserable. We wander from one project to the next looking for fulfillment, never filling the hole we feel deep inside. Even those who have accomplished their concoctions with great success—successful movie stars, politicians or CEOs of multinational corporations—remain unfulfilled. How do we know this? Because they keep looking for fulfillment. Once they have reached their lofty goals and dreams, it still wasn't enough. They are still empty inside.

The mind also becomes conditioned to the things we allow our body to do. Its programming is set up to continue on a particular track until the self pushes it off the track. This is especially true if the mind accomplishes even a little positive feedback from the body or self that what the body is doing is pleasurable.

This is a type of addiction—and it is why people become addicted. When the body partakes in an activity that stimulates the release of dopamine and/or endorphins among the brain and nerve cells, a feedback system is created that stimulates the mind's attachment to that activity. Why does the mind become attached? Because the inner self has the false assumption that the body is the self (false ego), the mind is programmed to consider any positive physical feedback as delivering on the self's intention for pleasure and/or love.

Sensual inputs stimulate dopamine and/or endorphins. These include visual inputs, tastes, aromas, music, tickling and other sensations to the skin, and a variety of physical activities including sex. Of course, those activities that require little effort to release the endorphins are favored. For example, lots of 'feel good' endorphins are released after a hard workout. But a hard workout requires, well, hard work.

Once the mind gets positive feedback from the brain cells in the form of dopamine and/or endorphins, that activity is now cemented into the mind as a "go to" concoction. Whenever the self is looking for fulfillment (which it perpetually is) the mind quickly inserts that activity as a concoction for the body to obtain. These "go to" concoctions, over time, shape our consciousness. The mind will focus upon those concoctions the self approves, and those that deliver some sort of positive physical feedback, regardless of whether they serve the greater purpose of the body or the self, will capture our attention.

As the mind programs the body to accomplish each successive concoction, it also facilitates innumerable sub-programs — or sub-concoctions. These are also ultimately intended to facilitate accomplishing the central intentions of the inner self. These sub-programs can range from training the body to accomplish specific strengths and functionality, to facilitating the body's autonomic reactions. These also include sub-features such as pulling the hand away from a fire to avoid losing the hand. If the hand is lost, many of the primary concoctions of the mind will be hindered. These sub-routines are developed with the self's ultimate goals in mind, and they accomplish the tasks of basic survival. These tasks have been categorized as *instinct.*

Biologists like to consider survival activities as instinctive, since many species seem to inherently seek survival with similar techniques. These are simply sub-routines of the mental concoctions to keep the body alive, however. This can be seen in cases where children were raised by animals — called *feral children.* As the syndrome — *Mowgli syndrome* – goes, the child turns out emulating the chief caregiver — be that an animal or handicapped parent. The mind of the child develops concoctions and sub-concoctions based on the perceptions and choices made available through association with those in the immediate family or group. This is also applicable to a child trained in a military school, or even in a terrorist camp-school. Each will come out with dramatically different strategies to achieve pleasure and love.

As the body's activities are driven by the mind's concoctions, its metabolic activities are orchestrated together with the routing of sensual inputs, memory, and feedback. The body can thus be said to be shaped by the mind's programming. The mind does not create the body, as is proposed by some. The body's functions are shaped and steered by the mind, however. The mind has the ability to direct the body to attempt to achieve its particular concocted strategies. We can also say that without that direction the body would probably not have achieved that result. However, the mind does not create or control the outcome. The mind has severe restrictions.

This conclusion can be arrived at scientifically. Despite our desire to, the mind cannot control the weather. The mind cannot control what others say. The mind cannot control the outcome of events. Attractive semantics used by some self-help "gurus" will claim that the only reason the mind may not control the outcome is due to some defect of thinking. Where is the defect of thinking when the weather is boiling hot or freezing cold and there is no ability to get out of this circumstance? Despite our mental attempts to change the weather, we simply cannot. Yes, we can pack our bags and travel to a better location. This decision will come at a cost, however. The mind cannot control these consequences. The next location is likely to also have its weather problems as well. The mind simply cannot change certain physical realities.

Mental Escape

The mind also cannot avoid trauma. Does the mind create the trauma of rape or other physical abuses? Is there some defect in the mind that has somehow attracted that event to the person—as the law of attraction proposes? This is not only an absurd notion, but it is cruel. Its implication is that all the suffering in the world is caused by our mental derangement.

Rather, traumatic events are learning experiences. The outcome is dependent upon whether the inner self learns what the trauma is supposed to teach. The body may be experiencing a particular traumatic event. However, the inner self only experiences the trauma to the extent the self is connected with the body and has committed to those related concoctions. If the self can release from these concoctions and detach from the mind's strategies, the trauma will heal because the inner self will have redirected the mind and body with new intentions.

We can either grow or shrink from trauma. This is our choice—the inner self has the power to make changes in direction. This is called intelligence. Therefore, continuing traumas are symptomatic of a lack of change despite life teaching us to change. Why is this? Simply because life was designed—actually programmed—by the Almighty to teach us to grow and progress through this lifetime, towards our higher purpose.

Why are some of us experiencing more trauma than others? In reality, every body experiences traumatic events. It is our lack of preparation for the event that makes it traumatic. For this reason, even unexpected loud sounds can become traumatic for a person who is not expecting the sound. This is referred to as *acoustic shock.*

The particular traumas we face depend upon our prior decisions and activities. Actions that inflicted cruelty or pain upon others will return reciprocal traumatic reactions either later in this life or into the next. This is the ultimate design of the universe.

In family psychology, there is a form of discipline called *learning by consequence.* This is described as a child being given specific consequences related to specific actions rather than unrelated punishment such as spanking. By design, our decisions and actions result in precise consequences—our current situation thus perfectly mirrors a combination of our current consciousness and what we have done in the past.

This reality has been confirmed in many past life regression studies, as we will discuss in detail later. In many studies, subjects' current fears or dilemmas can be related precisely to an activity they took part in within a past embodiment. The experience of the trauma allows the self to work through the issue, and resolve it by making the appropriate changes. If the self committed suffering upon others in a previous life, it will have to work through a similar trauma in this life. Once the trauma is experienced, the self can potentially grow and develop from the experience. Having experienced that traumatic event, the prudent self makes a determination not to ever commit that experience upon another—knowing what it feels like.

This determination is often made regardless of whether the person consciously realizes that the trauma happened because of an action they took in the past. The inner self will understand this in a deeper way, however. Through the decision to not partake in that activity, we have essentially learned the lesson, which will automatically resolve the trauma.

If we do not adequately grow from a trauma, it will likely bear upon us as a conflict to resolve later. As such, following a traumatic event, some of us will negatively retain the memory of the trauma. Most will seek to escape or release from this disturbing web of traumatic events. Often these attempts only serve to exacerbate the issues, as the intent to escape the memory causes a resurfacing of the disturbing memory.

Nature's system is designed to face the self with a resolution with trauma. This can render a change in direction, resulting in growth and evolution. If that change does not take place, there will likely be a continuing disturbance, or at least a buried trauma, which will emerge later to be reckoned with.

An example illustrating this burying mechanism is the use of propranolol—a pharmaceutical drug developed in the 1950s for depression. Propranolol works by blocking the reception of epinephrine on beta-adrenergic nerve receptors. When the epinephrine receptors are blocked, the mind can better disengage from stress because the feedback-response channels through which the limbic system and prefrontal cortex operate are inhibited, temporarily disengaging parts of the neural memory net.

Recent research on propranolol has revealed an additional unintentional effect, however: Clinical results have indicated that a person can also more easily release from past physical or emotional traumas by taking propranolol. Researchers observing these effects have documented women able to release from rape trauma and soldiers able to release from battlefield traumas, for example.

This use of propranolol has become controversial. Many ethics scientists have protested that using a synthetic drug to remove or disconnect from past trauma interferes with the natural learning process inherent in nature's mechanisms of remembering and resolving historical traumas. They correctly propose that without this natural mechanism, our ability to grow and evolve is stunted.

Both sides of this issue certainly have respectable positions. No one likes to see someone else suffer from their particular traumas. Yet it is critical that we learn and grow from our experiences. The question here is whether propranolol—like alcohol and many other mind-altering drugs—simply delays the trauma from being worked through—the lack of which may cause a later unforeseen fall-out. In the case of alcohol, which is used by many to escape from reality through similar biochemical mechanisms, more damage is eventually done by the attempted escape.

While the alcoholic may wish the world will get better and problems will dissolve, the problems simply worsen. Family and friends of the alcoholic simply become increasingly hurt and disaffected, and during drunken rages, the alcoholic may damage these relationships and create more problems. This in turn only makes the situation worse. This situation is illustrated by the large populations of homeless alcoholics. These people choose to try to escape from life's traumas. Ironically, the escape only aggravates those problems, and they evolve into full-blown disasters. Instead of improving the situation by our escaping from it, the problematic situation worsens and the traumas will still need to be reconciled along with the need for physical withdrawal. The recovering alcoholic will then have to deal with the problems caused by the alcohol in addition to resolving the initial traumas.

We might compare this again to the computer. In the case of propranolol, the blocking of epinephrine's reception would be equivalent to shutting down the computer terminal in order to shield the operator from a virus that is occurring within the computer's software and data. The virus is still there. It will not resolve itself. Shutting off the terminal will only allow the virus to grow and destroy more data. The operator must face the virus by employing an antivirus. By turning off the terminal, the operator does nothing to solve the problem.

This is basically what we try to do with drinking, taking drugs, watching TV or otherwise getting lost in some other diversion. We want to release from the anxieties and stresses of this world. We want to disengage ourselves from the traumas of life: From our job, from a difficult relationship, or from tough family situations. Periodically, most of us need escape. However, some partake in destructive forms that not only delay the fixing of the problem: they also make things worse. Others will simply exercise or go for a walk in the woods for release. Still others might garden, go shopping or go to a movie.

These types of release all certainly might work temporarily. Chemical releases such as alcohol or drug use are based upon the blocking or modulating of synaptic neurotransmitters, which change the information pathways through the nerves. When the synaptic receptors are blocked by the introduction of alcohol into the system, the information transmissions are muted or blocked. This means the mind cannot gain access to the critical mapping information needed to recalibrate with physical reality. The mind becomes slightly disconnected with the body. This provides a temporary release. However, the self may also lose considerable control over the body, including many autonomic functions necessary to maintain health. As a result, there are multiple physiological disorders associated with alcoholism and drugs, including diabetes and neuropathy.

The ultimate solution to these complexities comes from facing the problems of life dead-on: Why am I unhappy? Why are others around me so unhappy? Why are there so many wars, starvation and suffering in this world? Why did my friend or family member die? Why do I have to die?

These problems require singular focus from the self: Solving the problems of life begins with understanding who we are. From there we need to understand our purpose in life. We need to know what will make us happy: What will make us fulfilled?

If the self engages the mind for these purposes, the mind can actually be quite productive.

Chapter Three

Living after Death

Clinical Death

Evidence concluding our identity as separate from the body has been presented by a number of respected medical researchers over the past four decades. With the advent of resuscitation and medical life-support technologies has come a proliferation of patients whose bodies have clinically died prior to resuscitation. Author and researcher Dr. Raymond Moody pioneered this research in the 1960s, and introduced us to the *Near Death Experience* (or NDE). Dr. Moody presented hundreds of cases documenting common experiences among patients who were declared clinically dead and later were resuscitated in hospital and urgent care facilities.

Dr. Moody's research reviewed a cross-section of thousands of cases of patients with a variety of religious and socioeconomic backgrounds. Dr. Moody discovered a common experience: The patient described separating from the body, and floats above it. They view the various resuscitation efforts taking place on their body. This is often followed by a visit with relatives and loved ones. Traveling at the speed of thought to their homes or remote locations, they describe trying in vain to communicate with their loved ones, but they are not heard.

After viewing loved ones, many subjects detailed being drawn into a darkened tunnel with a bright light at the end. At the end of the tunnel, many encountered a dazzling person whom they described as God or an angel of God. Their lives were played back in an instant. Some spoke with this Personality, who in many cases indicated it was not their time yet. Following this, they instantly returned to their body. This often coincided with the resuscitation of the body (Moody 1975).

Naturally, this research had its skeptics. A few questioned Dr. Moody's protocols such as patient selection and interviewing techniques. Dr. Moody's patients were collected as their cases were presented to him. This offered some but not complete randomness.

This protocol gap was quickly filled by Kenneth Ring, Ph.D. In a well-received, peer-reviewed study published in 1985, Dr. Ring randomly selected 101 patients who had experienced an NDE. By contrast, the 101 patients studied by Dr. Ring were chosen randomly to eliminate any bias, imagination, hallucination, inconsistency, and other elements possibly affecting the objectivity of their after-death experiences.

Of the 101 subjects who underwent clinical death, a third recalled out-of-body experiences, and a quarter recalled entering the darkness or tunnel with the light at the end. About 60% reported at least a positive, peaceful experience. Those NDE subjects whose death was the result of a suicide attempt experienced no tunnel or light. The suicide NDEs in this study experienced a "murky darkness" after feeling separated from their body, but did not proceed any further. The rest had little or no recollection of the experience (Ring 1985).

Ring's findings — though not in the exact same percentages — were substantiated by professor of medicine and cardiologist Michael Sabom, M.D. Dr. Sabom documented his research in a 1982 work called *Recollections of Death: A Medical Investigation.* There have been several other studies confirming NDE experiences as well (Blackmore 1996).

In one, Dr. Elisabeth Kübler-Ross documented a lengthy study covering over twenty thousand cases of clinical death in her 1991 book *On Life After Death* — confirming the same primary conclusions arrived at separately by Sabom, Moody and Ring.

Upon review of the other various explanations, it appears unlikely that any of the possible physical causes could suitably explain NDE. The only reasonable explanation is that the self is not the body. The sheer cross-section of people with this same experience provides too much variance to provide any other rational explanation. NDEs occur regardless of religious reverence, expectations, brain state, drug-administration, NDE awareness, or biochemical stimulation.

Additionally, when the researchers compared NDE out-of-body observations with hospital staff reports, they almost without exception confirmed the observations of NDE subjects — made from outside of a body clinically dead. While unconscious and with eyes closed, the patient could hardly be expected to observe those events — even if by subconscious hearing. This is evident from the detail of the NDE subject descriptions.

Nonetheless, a few skeptical researchers have suggested that some sort of paranormal experience is involved in NDE experiences. However, we must ask these skeptics: How rational it is to accept the radical notion of a paranormal experience yet not accept an out-of-body observation? Either scenario requires an independent observer. In either scenario, there must be an observer separate from the event (clinical death) that can view events and report those events once being resuscitated.

In all, more than 25,000 clinical deaths have undergone scientific evaluation. The sheer quantity of near death experiences provides clear evidence for the fact that the inner self is not subject to the death of the body. The body is a temporary vehicle. When it breaks down, the inner self must leave. Should it be resuscitated, the self may return. It is actually quite simple.

Out of Body Experiences

Remote viewing provides another piece of evidence confirming that the inner self has a life beyond the body. Remote viewing is the ability to observe something outside of the confines and restrictions of the body's senses. Remote viewing is quite similar to NDE because most NDE subjects float above their body after clinically dying and remotely view the room and those activities occurring around their clinically dead body. This is the quintessential out-of-body experience.

In addition, many heart surgery patients have accurately reported remotely viewing the operation while they were clinically unconscious and under complete anesthesia with their eyes and faces covered. In one case, a heart surgery patient floated above the body and watched the heart surgeon perform an unusual maneuver that looked like he was making flapping motions with his arms and elbows during the operation. After the patient awoke, he precisely detailed the entire operation—including the surgeon's flapping motions—to the hospital staff. They were amazed because no one outside of the surgical team could have known the doctor did this funny little maneuver.

For twenty-three years, the Stanford University Research Institute studied parapsychological phenomena (also termed PSI—after the Greek letter *psi*, or *psyche*) such as remote viewing with a grant from the United States government. Two physicists named Dr. Russell Targ and Dr. Harold Puthoff teamed up for much of this research, and they conducted controlled experiments under the watchful eye of the CIA.

Much of this top-secret research was not released to the scientific community due to its sensitivity to international security. Part of the research consisted of sealing talented subjects into guarded rooms with observers. From the sealed rooms, the subjects remotely viewed and described in detail events and locations thousands of miles away. Their viewing documented minute details of the locations, down to the current weather conditions. They described specific geographical facilities, the locations of specific buildings, and activities taking place—years before internet use was common.

The locations and specifics of these observations were controlled and confirmed as being otherwise unavailable to the viewer. Two particular viewers, Pat Price and Ingo Swann, were able to identify military installations around the world, including then-secret Soviet bases on the other side of the planet. They also accurately described weather conditions at the time of viewing. Other experiments included placing objects on a table in a remote room. From a sealed room located thousands of miles away, the remove viewers were able to describe the objects in detail, including their positioning and orientation (Puthoff and Targ 1981; Puthoff *et al.* 1981).

Other remote viewing experiments over the years have since confirmed that many of us have this ability to "see" things not within our physical sensory range. It has been found that many people leave their bodies during sleep. Moreover, it seems this skill can be developed. Targ and Katra (1999) describe being able to develop that skill by attempting to:

> "...*separate out the psychic signal from the mental noise of memory, analysis and imagination.*"

These controlled studies illustrate the existence of a seer existing outside of the realm of the physical senses and neurons of the brain. If seeing was merely a biochemical and physiological experience driven by a mixture of molecules and cells, then who is it that is able to see things beyond the physical range of the eyeballs? Who is seeing and describing things that are half way around the world?

The limitations of our physical senses have been well established by science. As humankind has progressed technologically, we continue to gain new information about things we previously did not perceive through our gross sense organs. This growing technical facility increasingly makes it clear that our physical senses only perceive a small portion of the vast spectra of waveforms around us. Outside of the gross physical spectrum lies the subtle spectrum, and outside this lies the *conscious spectrum*. Our physical eyes and physical instruments simply are not equipped to see into this spectrum. The spectrum of the conscious dimension is transcendental to physical sense perception.

Transmigration

Transmigration means to move oneself from one location to another. With respect to the relationship between the body and the inner self, to transmigrate means to move from one body to the next. Some also call this reincarnation.

The problem with the word reincarnation is that it has been overly misused and ill defined. Many people think this means that the "person" (defined as the body) becomes another "person." This of course is an illogical proposition. It is also not the same as transmigration. In transmigration, the transcendental inner self moves from one body to another, just as a person might get out of one car and get into another.

One of the most important points to make in this regard is the fact that each of us has been moving from one body to the next even during this present lifetime. Consider looking at your body when it was in grammar school. Now look at your current body (assuming you are not still in grammar school!) That little body looks sort of like your current body in terms of some of the facial features. But the entire body is different. The body you wear now is a completely different body. In other words, you, the inner self, has changed bodies. As the body has gradually replaced all of its cells and molecules, the entire body has changed. You have effectively transmigrated from one body to the next — from your grammar-school body to your adult body.

This transmigration continues throughout life. We might compare the situation to a waterfall. While the waterfall might look the same from one minute to the next, it contains completely different water molecules. The actual waterfall is different from one moment to the next.

The manner in which the body changes is based upon the condition of our mind and consciousness. Those things we — the inner self — are interested in are expressed through our mind and body. Once we condition our mind to particular things, the mind becomes attached. As the mind becomes attached, the body's cells and genes cooperate and form around the condition of the mind.

Thus the form and condition of the body is shaped around the attachments of the mind. We can see this through this lifetime. A person who likes to eat will gradually develop a body that is capable of eating a lot of food. A person who likes to swim will gradually develop a body that can swim very well.

Athletes refer to this as training. When they want to excel in a certain sport they will train for that sport. The focus of their mind is concentrated upon conditioning the body. This will change the shape of the body to excel in that particular sport.

This same mechanism also works between bodies. At the time of death, the condition of our mind and consciousness will determine the form of the next body the inner self inhabits.

This reality is confirmed by the vast amount of hypnotherapy research performed over the past twenty years by eminent scientists. The procedure, called *past-life regression*, was in part developed by Dr. Ian Stevenson, a medical doctor and professor of research at the University of Virginia, Department of Psychiatric Medicine. Over several decades of research, Dr. Stevenson put hundreds of subjects under clinical hypnosis, drawing from them a recall of a previous lifetime.

It is interesting how Dr. Stevenson's research began. Being a conservative psychiatrist and medical professor, Dr. Stevenson had no prior belief in the transmigration of the self. He did, however, as many of his colleagues and a vast amount of evidence, believe that hypnotherapy was an appropriate therapeutic tool for mental issues and post-traumatic stress syndrome. During the application of clinical hypnotherapy, one of Dr. Stevenson's patients began to recall—in detail and historical accuracy—a life they had lived before and could not have been aware of. After corroborating the information, Dr. Stevenson went about the task of clinically uncovering others' past lives through regression.

His research documented hundreds of subjects who detailed previous lifetimes as historical persons, describing events with a clarity and experience only possible from having lived personally in that situation. Dr. Stevenson and other scientists meticulously corroborated the accuracy of these details, and gradually developed a mountain of practical evidence for the transmigration of the self.

Though undoubtedly controversial, the research has been thoroughly peer-reviewed and corroborated. Over thirty scientific books and hundreds of scientific papers have been written to document studies by hypnotherapists, many of whom are M.D.s and/or licensed psychiatrists. Dr. Stevenson's research spanned over thirty-seven years, and documented hundreds of cases of previous life recognition by children who remembered their past lives. His corroborated research indicated that past life recollection fades by about age seven. Before that age, children will often speak spontaneously about their previous lives as historical individuals, recalling historical details decades old and otherwise unknowable. Dr. Stevenson and his various associates meticulously documented these recollections along with the confirmations of their historical accuracy. Dr. Stevenson wrote several books on the subject, presenting the evidence in a clinically rigorous and scientific manner (Stevenson 1997; Tucker 2005).

As mentioned, a number of other scientists have documented regressing patients into verifiable past lives, including Dr. Helen Wambach (1978), Dr. Morris Netheron (1978), Dr. Edit Fiore (1978), Dr. Bruce Goldberg (1982), Dr. Joel Whitton (1986), Dr. Brian Weiss (1988), Dr. Christopher Bache (1994), Dr. Winafred Lucas (1993), Dr. Marge Rieder (1995; 1999) along with a number of others.

One of the more interesting studies was led by Dr. Rieder. She initially documented regression sessions with a number of patients that revealed historical information regarding Millboro, VA—a pivotal village during the Civil War. These subjects accurately described many historical and little-known details of the war and the town, details that were corroborated historically. The subjects had no other way of knowing those details. For example, many of the subjects described the use of a number of interconnected tunnels and hideaways in Millboro used during the war. Prior to the hypnosis regression, many of these tunnels and hideways were not known even by historians. The regression detailed the precise location of the tunnels, leading the researchers to discover them for the first time since the war.

To this, we can add the research of Dr. Michael Newton, a psychologist and master hypnotist who regressed patients into the period between their last body and the current body. Dr. Newton's patients consistently tell of inter-life judgment scenarios, karma and other topics in his 1994 *Journey of Souls: Studies of Life between Lives,* and his 2000 work, *Destiny of Souls: New Case Studies of Life between Lives.* Dr. Newton was a clinical specialist in pain management who stumbled onto the reality of past-lives while treating patients. His texts document some fifteen years of clinical research, and empirically illustrate the transitional ("judgement day") phase that exists after the death of this body.

The Ancient Knowledge

Prior to 2,000 years ago, transmigration of the self was a standard teaching among most of the ancient religions and philosophies. This of course included the Vedic and Buddhist philosophies. But it also included the Egyptians, Mayans, American Indians, Aboriginals and many others. All of the great religions understood transmigration of the self as a basic tenet of their philosophy. The Greeks, Romans, and Northern Europeans also assumed this philosophy — as did the Hebrew religion prior to the period of King Constantine and successors — who oversaw the politically-driven Synods of Nicea of the fourth century on. These specifically banned the teachings of transmigration of the self as put forth by early fathers of the Christian church such as Origen of Alexandria.

Origen Adamantius (185-254 A.D.) was a devout Christian scholar and minister who was a close associate of the Bishop of Alexandria. Origen had a flourishing school in Alexandria during the third century. He was considered one of the fathers of the early Christian church for several centuries. Consistent with the conclusions in this book, Origen taught that the self was spirit in essence, and transcendental to the body. Origen taught that each of us initially fell from God's grace by choice and took on a physical body. Once within the physical plane, the spiritual self then descends through the species, taking on one body after another, until again rising back to the human form of life. Here in the human form, Origen taught, we have the rare opportunity to return to God — should we use this human form wisely.

Should we make some progress but not enough, Origen taught, we may take on another human form until we progressed (evolved) to the level of returning to the spiritual world.

However, if we got caught up in the chase for animalistic pleasures — eating, sex, etc. — we may once again fall into the animal forms to again transmigrate between countless physical forms until we have another chance in the human form. This, Origen taught, was equivalent to hell.

There is a substantial amount of evidence that Jesus also taught the transmigration of the self. The Gnostic books of the Essenes, a society that Jesus lived in, support this, and even some of the four gospels of the New Testament indicate this possibility. For example, we find in the New Testament (NIV) that Jesus' disciples asked this question about a blind man:

> *"Rabbi, who sinned, this man or his parents, that he was born blind?"* (John 9:1)

Let's consider carefully the question. Why did Jesus' disciples ask this question? First we should consider that multiple disciples asked this question and not just one 'rogue' disciple. This means that it was a question that arose from an understanding between Jesus and his disciples from other teachings. In other words, it was assumed that before the man was born, he had the *ability* to sin. In other to have the ability to sin, the man must have had a previous physical body. Why? Because as Jesus taught previously, sinning was an action brought upon by the flesh. In other words, the person must have had a prior physical body in order to have sinned before he was born.

Note also that Jesus did not ridicule or criticize this question. He took it in stride. He did not say, "what a preposterous question." What he said was:

> *"Neither this man nor his parents sinned, but this happened so that the work of God might be displayed in his life. As long as it is day, we must do the work of Him who sent me."* (John 9:2)

Because Jesus accepted the question and answered it in acknowledgement that the man could have sinned before being born (just as the parents could have sinned) to cause his blindness, there was another purpose to the blindness. Still, this does not negate the fact that both Jesus and his disciples accepted the transmigration of the self as a matter of course.

We can add to this that Origen was a famous and devout person who dedicated his life to Jesus. In the end he became a martyr for his devotion to Jesus and God. Origen received the teachings of Jesus through his father, Leonides, a devoted Christian teacher who was also persecuted for his determined faith in God. There is good reason to believe that Origen's teachings were directly in line with one of Jesus' disciples. Origen was one of the most prolific Christian writers and well-known Christian teachers of that era, with possibly thousands of students at his Catechetical School of Alexandria, where Clement of Alexandria had also instructed. Origen's teachings were also supported by the bishops Alexander of Jerusalem and Theoctistus of Caesarea of that time, and he had a close personal relationship with Demetrius, the Bishop of Alexandria. Origen was a devoted Christian who gave personal care for thousands of imprisoned Christians. He was a prolific writer, and his commentaries and translations of scriptures were well respected throughout the region. He is said to have produced some 6,000 writings during his lifetime. In one, Origen wrote:

> Or is it not more in conformity with reason, that every soul, for certain mysterious reasons is introduced into a body, and introduced according to its deserts and former actions? It is probable, therefore, that this soul also, which conferred more benefit by its former residence in the flesh than that of many men (to avoid prejudice, I do not say "all"), stood in need of a body not only superior to others, but invested with all excellent qualities. (*Against Celsus*, I.32)

Certainly the dedication and passion Origen had for serving God and Jesus, and his acceptance by the early church indicates that he wouldn't have simply made up the philosophy of the transmigration of the self without a strong foundation of scripture. Origen in fact was highly committed to scripture as having ultimate authority, and all of his writings quoted scriptural passages. These facts all add up to one certain notion: That the transmigration of the soul was embraced by many in the early Christian church in the second century after Jesus' disappearance. Are we to deny the possibility that it was also part of Jesus' teachings as well?

Everything changed in the fourth century. In 325 A.D. and periodically thereafter, Constantine and his successors organized the Hebrew/Christian church and dictated its teachings through the legislation of the Synods of Nicea. Here bishops of different regions were brought together into a politically oriented committee to produce a unilateral interpretation of the Jewish faith and Christianity. These and other governmental decrees resulted in massive restrictions on what could be taught within the Hebrew and Christian world. These culminated in an insidious persecution of anyone involved in teaching the transmigration of the self—which has continued (though less violently) through modern times. Evidence of this is found in the Fifth Ecumenical Council of Constantinople, as it pushed forth this official anathema (meaning "to banish") against Origen and similar teachers:

> "If anyone does not anathematize Arius, Eunomius, Macedonius, Apollinaris, Nestorius, Eutyches and Origen, as well as their impious writings, as also all other heretics already condemned and anathematized by the Holy Catholic and Apostolic Church, and by the aforesaid four Holy Synods and if anyone does not equally anathematize all those who have held and hold or who in their impiety persist in holding to the end the same opinion as those heretics just mentioned: let him be anathema."
> (5th Ecumenical Council: Constantinople II, 553)

We notice here that other great teachers are also being banished together with Origen. These include Nestorius, who was the Archbishop of Constantinople in the fifth century; and Apollinaris, who was either Apollinaris Claudius, Bishop of Phrygia or Apollinaris of Laodicea, the Bishop of Laodicea (Syria).

The ancient traditions of gnosis, hermeticism and hellenism, which descended through the Greek texts from antiquity inclusive of ancient Egyptian teachings, also taught transmigration. Hermes Trismegistus, revered amongst Christian, Islam and Jewish sects, is said to have stated:

> *"O son, how many bodies have we to pass through; how many bands of demons; through how many series of repetitions and cycles of the stars; before we hasten to the One alone?"*

We also find this passage, translated from ancient sermons and fragments of later Trismegistic literature (Mead 1906):

> *"What then is the value nowadays of that ancient doctrine mentioned by Plato, about the reciprocal migration of souls; how they remove hence and go thither, and then return higher and pass through life. And then again depart from this life, made quick again from the dead? Some will have it that this is a doctrine of Pythagoras, while Albinus will have it to be a divine pronouncement, perhaps of Egyptian Hermes."*

There is also evidence that the teaching was accepted by the original teachings of the Koran:

> *"How can ye reject the faith in Allah? Seeing that you were without life, and He gave you life; then will He cause you to die, and will again bring you to life; and again to Him will you return."* (Al-Baqara 2:28)

Today, transmigration of the self is most often considered an Eastern religious philosophy, along the lines of the Buddhist or Hindu faiths. These teach almost an identical description of transmigration as that taught by Origen and Hermes. Here the self is also described as a transcendental spiritual entity transmigrating from one body to the next. As the self evolves, it takes on progressively higher forms until the human form is achieved. In the human form, according to the most ancient Vedic texts, the self has an opportunity to return home to God and the transcendental world. Should the self be caught in the 'wheel' of karma, it may be dragged once again down into the lower forms of life.

Should the self become reconnected with God by way of devotional service, the self may transcend the physical body. Should the self make some progress but not reach perfection, it may take on another human form. Here again, there is the risk that the attachment to the physical world may return the self to taking on bodies of lower forms of life. These include animals, fish, insects and even plants, according to the Vedas — the world's oldest theistic scriptures.

The Evolution of the Self

This leads us to the concept of the self's evolution. In order to rise to the point of the human form of life, one's consciousness must be at that state of evolution.

This mechanism also correlates — with limitations — with the observations that led to the evolution theory put forth by Darwin and many others since. Certainly we can see how all the creatures of the earth seem to be related to each other somehow. How does this seeming evolution of physical bodies relate to the self's evolution to the human form? Perhaps we should start by discussing the modern evolutionary theory, and its limitations.

The evolutionary theory has dominated biological sciences for over one hundred years. This theory has also been the subject of intense debate over that period, primarily because it conflicts with certain religious teachings.

The debate has become intense. Those who have faith in the Biblical version have been accused as lacking scientific credibility. Evolutionary theorists have been accused of having no faith in God. For many years the two camps argued aggressively, and no end appears in sight. Over the last few years some have proposed a version of creation and evolution that assumes the existence of God — called intelligent design. This theory has been met with debate from both ends. The Biblical camp says intelligent design conflicts with the Bible. The evolutionists have proposed that intelligent design does not adequately answer the need for empirical evidence.

The original evolutionary theory of Darwin has been revised over the years to accommodate recent research on genetics. It has been combined with the assumption of a chemical basis for life—which some refer to as the *primordial soup theory*. Most recently, the evolutionary theory has been revised to include the concept of epigenetics.

The concept of evolution stands up to the test of credibility in many ways when it comes to physical evidence and observation. There is also some carbon dating that also confirms the existence of humanity as well as other creatures millions of years ago—far outdating a literal chronology of the Bible.

However, there are some fundamental problems with the theory of evolution. The first lies with the underlying premise of an accidental beginning and continued randomness among the evolutionary course. According to the basic theory, every creature supposedly evolved from the accidental and spontaneous birth of a single living unicellular organism. This we discussed earlier. This original organism theoretically became more complex incidentally through the processes of *genetic mutation, survival of the fittest* and *natural selection.*

Fossil evidence and diversity among species certainly present a compelling case for the progressive improvement of certain species. Breeding observations also show that mutations develop through generations. Still there are some weaknesses in the theory. There is little evidence of any genetic connection between humans and dinosaurs, for example. Yet the assumptions of the theory would necessitate that these life forms were either ancestors of humans, or at the very least, cousins. The other critical problem, as we illustrated scientifically in the first chapter, is the sheer improbability of all the mutations necessary for the evolution from a single cell to a human within a few hundred million years occurring *accidentally.*

This truly fantastic assumption of the spontaneous creation of life assumes that chemicals somehow developed the *desire* to survive. Chemicals somehow developed the intention to improve their chances of survival. Have we ever observed chemicals desiring survival? Chemicals simply do not display this characteristic. No scientist has ever found the intent to survive outside of a living organism. No chemical moves towards survival without being part of a living organism. Chemicals may react and form various substances, and certainly will change structure when heated or cooled. Having a desire to survive is another matter altogether.

The desire to survive is connected to the desire to improve survival factors and eliminate threats to survival. The need to improve survival requires that *someone* values survival. This would require chemicals valuing their existence somehow, which in turn requires the chemicals to somehow recognize a difference between living chemicals and dead chemicals. This in turn requires that chemicals have awareness, because the desire to survive requires an awareness of self-existence. It also requires a fear of death—an illogical consciousness for a chemical.

In other words, in order to desire to survive, a living organism must be aware, consciously or subconsciously, that it is alive. A living organism must be able to differentiate itself from others and other chemicals. If there is no distinction between life and lifeless chemicals, why avoid death? Why desire life without a distinction between living and nonliving chemicals? Certainly it would be easier for a batch of chemicals to remain dead chemicals than to struggle for survival in the midst of all the environmental challenges to remain living.

A small unicellular organism could be killed by so many environmental challenges: freezing, direct sun exposure and any number of natural enemies. If there were no distinction between living or dead chemicals, then the path of least resistance would be to remain dead chemicals. If there were no awareness and desire for survival in the face of all this resistance, no living creature would bother to avoid death. This in turn would mean no incentive for survival—the opposite premise for evolution.

Put more simply, if a living entity could not distinguish itself from a nonliving entity there would be no urge to survive. Without the urge to survive, there would be no motivating factor to encourage adaptation or mutation. There would be no impetus to evolve because survival is not valuable without an awareness of life.

From a scientific view, an accidental and incidental evolution of bodies irrespective to the living beings within those bodies simply has no logical basis. An organism cannot desire to survive without an inner self or consciousness. This inner self or consciousness is what spurs the improvements that take place within the body. With no desire to survive, there is no adaptation to threats to survival.

It is only when the self values survival that the physical body could possibly learn to adapt to environmental factors. In fact, each physical body shape is specifically reflective of the condition of the consciousness of the inner self. It is not as if the inner self is within the body of a wolf, while its consciousness is more like a mouse. No. The wolf body reflects the inner self's consciousness. The body is not evolving in the evolution process: It is the inner self who is evolving. Each body is designed to reflect the evolution of the inner self occupying that body.

This is supported by a plethora of evidence. In the 1950s, a fox breeding experiment directed by Dr. Dmitry Belyaev of the then-Soviet Union's Institute of Cytology and Genetics in Novosibirsk studied mutation in breeding. The intent of this forty-year long study was to determine the genetic role humans played in the domestication of animals, particularly dogs, which theoretically evolved from foxes and wolves over the improbable period of ten thousand years. Most importantly, Dr. Belyaev wanted to study how contact with humans might bring about new behavior and changes in body features and physiology. The prime subjects of the study were silver foxes, who were cruelly caged while they and their offspring were put through various degrees of contact with humans.

The results were revealing. After over thirty generations of foxes were handled and petted by humans, profound changes became apparent when compared to undomesticated controls. One of the most apparent physical changes was the development of droopy ears among the domesticated foxes. Rather than the perky upright ears seen among wild wolves and foxes, these domesticated foxes developed floppy ears. One cannot help but be reminded of the sight of domesticated killer whales, who also mysteriously tend to develop floppy dorsal fins during their cruel capture and domestication in public aquariums.

Other observed effects of domestication include the fact that domestic foxes developed rolled up tails rather than tails pointing straight up. This appears analogous to the floppy ear characteristic. Dr. Belyaev speculated that the pointed ears and tails were possibly used by the foxes both as defense (to stand tall against challengers) and to sense the external environment more acutely. During captivity within protective dens provided by humans, these facilities were no longer necessary for survival.

Other significant differences were seen among neurotransmitter and hormone biochemistry. The domesticated foxes had significantly higher levels of serotonin in the bloodstream, and their corticosteroids would cycle differently than their wild relatives.

Behavioral changes were also consistently observed as the foxes became domesticated. Over generations, they became increasingly relaxed and comfortable around humans, responding positively to petting and other touching. Their ability to respond and communicate with humans also increased over the generations.

When we consider the central difference between the domesticated environment and the undomesticated environment of Dr. Belyaev's fox studies, the central difference outside the possibility of attack was being in the company of an organism (humans) of higher consciousness. If we consider that at least part of the physical and behavior alterations were specifically related with the rate of being in the proximity and care (and protection) of humans, then we must logically connect their genetic and behavioral changes with their proximity to organisms of higher consciousness. Instead of having to defend themselves in the wild, the foxes were protected and fed daily.

This encouraged the foxes to see the humans as advocates. As the foxes gradually got closer to humans, and began relating with their human handlers through touch and behavior, they began to trust the humans. As a result, their behavior and physical features changed because they learned to rely upon the humans. This was accompanied by biochemical changes and epigenetic changes. This is also consistent with an animal of one species being raised by another species. There are behavioral and physical changes resulting from a relationship between conscious individuals.

Consider for a moment how our bodies can also change and adapt with our changing desires, activities, and relationships. A long-distance runner who trains and races for several years will most likely become slender with well-built calves and thighs. These developments, along with better-conditioned lungs, give the runner an edge over the untrained runner. These changes will be accompanied by subtle genetic changes that govern metabolic responsiveness. On the other hand, a person who tends to overeat will probably develop a larger stomach, enabling more eating. Assuming a lack of exercise, this will likely accompany the creation of more fat cells and corresponding genetic changes, possibly including surtuin-related sequence alteration.

The changes in our current physical body are a result of our intentions, decisions and past activities. This is the design of the physical world. The shape of the body will reflect our choices in life: This is a net change due to consciousness. Should we decide to become a boxer, for example, we will likely end up with a broken or twisted nose and a puffy, scarred face. Likewise, a hardened violent criminal will probably have a number of scars and injuries because of his or her choices. An accountant, on the other hand, will probably have more delicate physical features. He or she will likely have smaller, weaker muscles as a result of their intentional choices and subsequent activities. Though we can easily connect stronger muscles with more exercising, the determination to exercise arose from an intentional self.

We can easily see how our physical features reflect our consciousness in so many different ways. Our current consciousness is the combination of our current desires and our past behavior.

We can see how our current status reflects decisions we have made in this lifetime or decisions we made in a past lifetime. As our consciousness changes, so does our body. We can scientifically and logically conclude that our various bodies (and species) reflect our evolving consciousness.

This brings us to the real problem of evolution. There is no consideration of the unique consciousness residing within each body. Where did this consciousness come from? Evolution is based upon an erroneous assumption that there is no distinct living driver within each physical body: It assumes that we are all simply physical machines without unique individuality, and without an existence outside of the body. This is inconsistent with the evidence, as we have reviewed in detail.

Every human, animal, fish, insect and plant maintains a unique desire to survive and adapt against the odds. Even the smallest of organisms, including single-celled paramecia have illustrated conscious behavior, with problem-solving abilities and an individual desire to survive.

In order to appropriately understand our past and the past of other living organisms, we must be able to view it within the context of the living portion of the organism. If we accept that each living organism contains a unique spark of consciousness, the discussion of evolution without a consideration of this individual consciousness would be akin to proposing that the earth is populated by walking chemical robots.

We might also study the development and evolution of trains over the last 100 years. We could describe how they mechanically evolved from the old coal-fired trains into electric speed trains. However, without a consideration of the engineers and builders who designed, built and ran them; and the executives and politicians who financed and promoted the industry, we would be ignoring the functional elements within the evolution of trains. The evolution of train type and performance were the result of many individuals who drove design and performance forward. The trains did not evolve by themselves.

Each living organism contains a unique personality, complete with independent feelings, emotions, desires and the need to love and be loved. It is essential this living element not be ignored. As we record and recall human history, we focus upon those historical persons that advanced human knowledge or achievement. We don't ignore the living personalities who spurred humanity's progress forward.

Thus we find that the best historians will focus upon the personal and emotional issues of historical persons. This is because they recognize that behind their accomplishments was a unique personality who made certain choices in life. It is not as if historical events just randomly occurred. There were made by personalities with unique emotions and talents.

Similarly, as we look back at the history of life on earth, we must recognize that behind each species are individuals who drove the evolution of that species. They also—down to every plant and cell—desire love. This desire drives the mating process, which expands the population of species. Mating is an activity of every living organism. Most organisms protect their offspring with vigor. Why such a vigor to protect another, even at the expense of ones own safety? Certainly a species with minimum intelligence has no motive to continue or enlarge the species. The prime motivation for mating and parenting among all living organisms is the quest for love. This is because within every creature is a spiritual being with an innate need for love.

In the 1960s, a group of psychologists (Harlow 1962; 1964; 1965) cruelly studied the relationships between monkeys and their mothers. Some baby monkeys were cruelly pulled away from their mothers at birth and put in isolated cages. The scientists observed that these monkeys quickly became hostile, depressed, and unstable as compared with caged monkeys united with their mothers.

Some of the baby monkeys were left alone with wire-built frames made to look like the shape of a monkey. Some of these frames were even built with milk-bottle breasts so the monkey could feed from a pair of fake nipples. Although the baby monkeys tried to hug the fake monkeys and suck milk from the fake breasts, they also became hostile, depressed, and unstable. They simply did not receive the gratification brought on by a loving relationship between mother and child.

Some of the monkeys isolated or caged with wire surrogates were introduced to live monkey surrogates who were not their mothers. These monkeys immediately began to hug the surrogates, and these stressed and hostile monkeys gradually became "normal" (for being cruelly imprisoned in cages).

The instinctive exchange of a loving relationship with another living being is critical to the existence of every living being. Once baby monkeys were allowed to exchange a relationship with a living being, they normalized. This is because every living being needs to exchange loving relationships. Contact with a physical form without a living being inside of it (like the monkey wire frames) will not replace our need for a relationship with a living being. The inner self needs to connect with another living being. If we were all physical machines, there would be no need for loving other living beings. We would be fully satisfied with lifeless robots and mannequins.

The case for our innate need for love is also made among human babies. Several peer-reviewed studies have compared preemie babies (preterm infants) who were held, stroked and/or massaged with preemies who were not. Preemie babies held more often and stroked or massaged, grew 47% faster; were significantly more alert; were less stressed and were more responsive to the world around them than preemies who were more isolated during incubation. The touched babies were also calmer and better adjusted later in their childhood than babies who were not touched as often (Field *et al.* 1986; Hayes 1998; Dieter *et al.* 2003). This result has been confirmed among lovingly stroked neonatal rats compared to those not stroked (Schanberg and Field 1987). Every organism hosts a love-seeking inner self.

The conclusion we can draw from this evidence is that it is not the species who have evolved over millions of years: It is the evolution of consciousness of associated living beings that has shaped the physical condition of each species.

Chapter Four

The Science of Faith

Most will consider this chapter heading an oxymoron. Can faith be scientific? As we'll discuss, there is quite a bit of scientific credibility for the belief in a Supreme Being. When looking objectively, in fact, a Supreme Being is a more scientific hypothesis than a universe that came into being from an accidental nuclear explosion. Let's investigate some of the tenets of faith from a scientific view.

Nirvana? Enlightenment?

The modern Buddhist philosophy teaches that if the self is successful in the human form of life, then after death, the living being either fades into "nothingness," or expands into "everything."

This philosophy proposes that the living being does not have an individual identity after death: Instead, the now individual self simply vanishes and evaporates into space—also called the void—or merging into "everything"—sometimes referred to as the white light. These assume that before death we are individuals, and after death we merge into a vast ocean of consciousness.

This does not meet with logic, nor is consistent with the research. Each of us is an individual; and clinical death, NDE and OBE research confirm that we remain individuals after the death of our body.

Each individual self must maintain a unique and distinct personality in order to conduct life within a body separated from others. Having an independent will stimulates activities that differentiate from others. This requires perpetual individuality. This individuality is expressed through our unique personalities. It is also expressed through the uniqueness between each of us. While we each wear a generally similar body, each of us have unique gene expression, unique fingerprints, unique talents, and a unique combination of cells, bacteria, metabolism and health issues.

These unique characteristics also point to an individual existence prior to birth, as confirmed by Dr. Stevenson's and others' work. If the self existed as an individual prior to birth and throughout a lifetime within a body that is constantly undergoing molecular and cellular change (ergo, a changing body), is it logical that the self would lose its individuality after the ultimate body change — death?

The Buddhists propose that when the inner self has evolved to a point of perfection, it can become one with the universe. This is not actually what Buddha taught. Buddha taught enlightenment, which is the realization of God or nirvana. In fact, after many attempts to attain the enlightenment as taught by local impersonalist teachers, Buddha condemned the methods of the rejection of the eternal self.

Yes, Buddhahood brings about the loss of the physical conception of life. But it does not negate our individual existence. In order to be enlightened, one must be an individual, separate from those who are not enlightened. In other words, if we were all one, how could some of us become enlightened while others were not? The logic of nirvana as fading into nothingness or everything is actually a misinterpretation of Buddha's teachings, which taught that once we gain enlightenment, we see our Buddha nature within — seeing the physical body as mere matter. The physical body becomes "nothing" to us, because we have become enlightened to our real spiritual existence.

> *"You say there is a void; therefore the void is not nothing; therefore there is not the void."*
> — Parmenides (5th century B.C.)

The inner self is the underlying source of our personality; our feelings, emotions, desires, the ability to love, and the desire to be loved. This personality is distinct from the mental programming taking place through the brainwaves and neural network of the physical body. Beyond the physical programming, each of us retains an independent, active inner self with a central objective of happiness, and receiving and giving love. Is it logical that this active being—continually seeking happiness and loving relationships—would suddenly abandon these propensities and permanently merge into a state of nothingness or mass consciousness?

What should the purpose of a temporary separate existence be then? Could a vague ocean of consciousness or nothingness separate into a multitude of individual purpose and will? Furthermore, the living self has maintained a consistent existence throughout many decades of a changing physical body. This equates to surviving a body that is continually dying. Does it seem logical that the fatal death of the same body would then remove our inherent will to survive and prosper? Should the death of this temporary body abruptly end our desire to love and exchange love?

Purpose and activity are the key distinctions between living and dead matter. Both of these elements (purpose and activity) indicate the existence of individuality. The very definition of *consciousness* requires individuality. Consciousness requires *awareness.* Awareness of something or someone requires individuality. Otherwise, there would be no one available to become aware, and nothing to become aware of. Logically, an "ocean of merged consciousness" would then be an oxymoron.

This of course is consistent with every other theistic religious philosophy. Once a person has evolved to the point where they re-connect with their spiritual nature, they can leave the body behind and enter the spiritual world. This is the "kingdom of God," "heaven," and so many other references to the spiritual world. This world is the home and origin of the inner self.

The tenth-century Vedic scholar Ramanuja explained the distinction between the spiritual world and the ocean of consciousness to be like a green bird entering a green forest. If we were looking from a distance at a green forest area, we would see a sea of green. If we then saw a green bird fly from next to us into this distant green forest, we might think the bird had merged into the green forest. We could make no distinction, from a distance, between the bird and the forest. They would appear to become one.

Yet we know, as Ramanuja explained, that the bird did not become the forest. We know the bird is still a bird despite having flown into the forest. If we walked into the forest, in fact, we would likely see the bird and many other birds like him. We would also see many different types of plants, flowers, trees and other creatures. Even though the forest looked like a sea of green from a distance, it actually is full of individuality and variegatedness. It is full of life, in other words.

Heaven is no different. While many teach that we will merge into nirvana or heaven when we die, this is not supported by science. Those who die and return to their bodies report that they continue to exist as individuals, and they are greeted 'on the other side' by other individuals. In other words, we each retain our individuality, regardless of whether we are inside the body or outside the body.

Our Need for Love

Every one of us is continually seeking someone to love and love us unconditionally. Loving relationships are our foremost focus from the time we are born into this physical body through to our leaving the body. As babies, we seek the attention and admiration of the people around us through physical contact, approval, and acceptance with other living beings. This drive for loving relationships via these external attempts continues throughout life, becoming the central rationale for our choice of mates, houses, cars, sports, careers, and so on.

People will sometimes endanger themselves to achieve the love of others. Some climb mountains or perform other death-defying feats to gain the attention and admiration (confused with love) of others. Due to the quest to achieve or maintain particular relationships, a person may put themselves in harm's way. Some may sacrifice their lives in a war while others may sacrifice money, an organ, or other material possessions on behalf of or in search of a loving relationship.

Love is held up in society as an aspiration every person should seek — the key to happiness. It is assumed that a successful loving relationship is the ultimate success in life. No one really understands why love has such a high priority, but most agree that those who love the most are also the happiest.

However, love cannot be accomplished alone. Love requires a lover and a beloved: a relationship. Love cannot exist without a loving relationship between at least two distinct and unique individuals.

This also means that the individuals must be separate enough to have the freedom to love each other. Love cannot be forced. This is slavery. Love can only exist when each individual has the choice to love the other.

True love is selfless and unconditional. Love is the caring of another without any expectation of a return. Loving someone is the act of humbly giving oneself to ones beloved. This type of true love will overwhelm all other aspects of ones life—minimizing one's self-regard.

This means that love is connected to service. Service is the ongoing expression of our love for another. Love without service is mere sentiment.

True love brings joy to both the beloved and the lover. True love is the food of the living being. We all need it because it is part of our constitutional nature: it is part of our true identity.

Every living being has an innate need to give oneself to another and to have the unconditional love of another upon oneself. That exchange of love; to serve and sacrifice oneself for a loved one, is aspired to throughout our society as the highest form of fulfillment. Each of us has tasted a small reflection of the joy of love to a minimal degree in one respect or another. Our acceptance of the importance of love in real life contradicts any chemical or evolutionary theories of love. Even the scientists who propose theories that love is a biochemical response still at the end of the day seek out love in their own personal lives. And even those who do not secrete these biochemicals well—such as those with Parkinson's disease—still seek loving relationships with others.

Every living being needs to exchange a loving and caring relationship with another living being. This is expressed among birds that care for their chicks; elephants that fend off for their fellow mates; dogs that pine to be stroked; and monkeys who hug and kiss other monkeys. Living beings have a fundamental, instinctual desire to be loved, to love and serve a beloved. This is the common universal trait of the living being. Regardless of race, creed, gender, or species, love is at the very core of our existence.

Although love is often characterized as an emotion, actually emotions stem from our desire for love. Love comes from a realm outside the gross physical dimension. Love transcends the temporary nature of the physical dimension because it is the very nature of the living being. Just consider the love for someone whose body has died. Does that love terminate when the body's life was terminated? Surely not. The love for that person continues, despite the status of their physical body. This illustrates the transcendental nature of love: It is not limited by the physical elements.

The living being cannot be separated from love. This is why people need other people to love. Without other living beings to exchange love with, we whither away in loneliness. This has been illustrated in studies that show that hospitalized patients live longer when they are attended to by family. The relationships within the family motivate the self to remain in the body.

We seek to exchange loving relationships with other living beings because love is a part of our constitutional nature. We are, in fact, creatures of love.

Since love is only expressed when one gives of oneself to another, love is not distinguishable from ones very being. When someone truly gives their love to another, they are giving the only thing they truly own—their decision to give of themselves. Every other possession is temporary to the living being. We know this scientifically because we can see that everyone leaves behind all their possessions at death. Since they leave behind those possessions, they never really owned them in the first place—since ownership must include control over the possession.

The ability to freely give our love, and choose where to put that love is the only thing we can take with us when our bodies die. Therefore, it is the only thing we own.

Where is Real Love?

Lust, greed and self-love are simply perverted forms of real love. Real love can only be expressed between two or more living beings. Some people speak of self-love as love but this is a perversion of love. Self-love is simply selfishness. It is diametrically opposed to love. When ones natural inclination to love is directed at oneself, this creates greed.

Real love is the act of humbly giving oneself to another living being. We cannot give ourselves to ourselves because we already have ourselves. There is nothing to give. Note that giving requires a giver, a gift (in this case love), and a receiver. The same person cannot be both the giver and the receiver because the gift has to change hands in order to be given. Therefore, self-love is merely selfishness and greed dressed up in seductive language.

We are never completely satisfied with this perverted form of love within the physical dimension. This is evidenced by the many relationships supposedly based upon love that evolve into break-up, divorce or loathing. These so-called relationships of love can also end in bitterness and anger. Why would they end this way if they were truly based upon love?

In reality, most of the relationships of the physical world are simply business deals. They are two (or more) people who have been brought together by mutual desires. In other words, they help each other accomplish their desires. The expressions of love in these relationships are simply given in order to receive something in return. This type of exchange is not love. It is business. These expressions might appear loving, but they are simply self-centered. They are grounded in each party's desire to receive or consume something for themselves.

There may even be a small tinge of real love mixed in with these 'business' relationships, but the desire to get something in return virtually drowns out those tinges. Even service performed in the name of this physical love/greed exchange is typically not given in love. It is usually performed to receive some benefit now or down the road.

Sincere love will only occur in connection with our transcendental existence. Love is part of our spiritual constitution. If we accept that love is the deeper and necessary aspect of our being, and we agree that our ultimate identity lies beyond the physical dimension, we must recognize that there is a living source of love beyond this physical dimension. After all, how could an emotion that is specifically exchanged between living beings not originate from a living being? Since love requires a lover and beloved, this source of love must also be able to exchange love.

Moreover, since the source of something must contain its ultimate nature, the source of love must be an ultimate lover and beloved. It is like two parents conceiving. This new baby is alive due to its parents being alive. According to one of the oldest rules of physics: organized energy must have an outside organizing force. Nothing comes from nothing. As Socrates and many others have elaborated, the ideals of love in this universe must logically have a permanent source outside the temporary physical dimension.

The very fact that we search throughout our lives for the ultimate loving relationship to complete ourselves indicates we know deep within that an unconditional lover and beloved exists. Since we are perpetually seeking unconditional love here without finding it, there must logically be someone who can receive and exchange that love. Why else would we strive so hard with the expectation that we will find someone who loves us unconditionally?

Love is at the very core of our being. It is the essence of our existence. We seek a loving relationship in order to feel complete. We cannot deny this either scientifically or practically. Anyone who has "fallen in love" will tell us that they felt more complete after they found this person. Unfortunately, the unconditional nature of their love was an illusion, evidenced by the fact that every one of these relationships end in breakup, divorce or at the very least, mutual aggravation and compromise. We realize in the end that they are not the perfect person we hoped they would be. If we are lucky, we can settle for a relationship of mutual respect and friendship—maybe even with some conditional love mixed in.

All of this points to the existence of a person outside the physical dimension with whom we can exchange an unconditional loving relationship. Our need for someone to love is not just anyone. Rather, the person we are seeking is no common person. We are looking for our perfect soul mate: A person who is always forgiving and understanding. Someone who would never lie or be deceitful to us. A person who is always be attractive to us and would never die on us. For this reason, many of us will often say our true love "is out there somewhere."

Our expectation of our true love or soul mate seems too good to be true. Or is it? Perhaps there is a perfect person "out there" after all. Logically, a perfect person must be able to control their environment. A perfect person could not be subject to the fallibilities typical among us humans. Who could have this sort of infallibility but the Supreme Living Being? Who could maintain the perfection of unconditional love other than the origin of love? Who could offer us complete shelter and trust other than the person who knows us the best? Someone who created us, perhaps? Our closest relative? We could not be talking about anyone other than God, could we?

Where is Heaven?

Heaven has been presented to us by spiritual wise men and saints for thousands of years. Heaven's existence has been documented in every theistic scripture of the world. Even still, there is great controversy and speculation about heaven and its location. Why is this?

It is due simply to a lack of trust in those who have already presented heaven to us. While faith is often thought of as joining a particular religious sect or denomination, the real definition of faith is trust: Do we trust what the great saints such as Abraham, Moses, Solomon, David, Jesus, Mohammad, Ramanuja, St. Francis, Vyasadev and many others have written or spoken about heaven? Or do we simply want to speculate?

Here we will present neither speculation nor a sectarian position. We will simply provide the position that is consistent with all the great teachings of saints from every monotheistic discipline. Here are seven key principles to consider:

First Principle: God is the Original Being and the Creator. God created everything in existence, including us.

Second Principle: God is the All-Powerful Being. He controls every part of His creation. Never is He out of control. God never comes under the illusion of the physical universe. He created the physical universe and its illusions. This means that God does not become subject to the laws of the physical universe. God does not lose control of His creation because He is God.

Third Principle: Rebellious living beings like ourselves are given temporary physical bodies as vehicles of learning. Within the body dwells a spiritual being—each of us are individual spiritual beings. When we are dwelling in the physical world, we are not our physical bodies. This does not mean that we do not have a body. We each have a spiritual body, but our spiritual body is non-different from our self. God also has a Body. His Body is spiritual, and thus non-different from Himself.

Fourth Principle: The spiritual world is a universe transcendental to the physical world. At the same time, heaven is anywhere where God's will is being done. Since God has created everything, and owns everything, the distinction between heaven and hell is that heaven is where God's will is being done, and hell is where God's will is not being done. In those places where God's will is not being done there is typically greed, hatred, jealousy, violence and pain. This is because selfishness is the driver of this dimension. In God's dimension—where His will is done—there is love, compassion, peace, giving, and devotion. In God's dimension there is no selfishness, because everyone there is in love with God. This love for God naturally spreads to all of God's children as well. As a result, everyone in God's dimension is working hard to take care of God and take care of others. This is because God is a nice God. He is a caring God. He wants us to naturally love Him because that is why He created us—to exchange a loving relationship with Him. (Why else would God have created us? Everyone—even God—needs a playmate, friend and lover.) In the spiritual dimension, time does not exist. Since time does not exist there, none of the rules governing the physical relationships of distance, speed, age and death apply. Like the physical universe, there are a variety of different locations and environments within the spiritual universe. Different living beings inhabit those different locations. We each have a particular relationship with the Supreme Person, and our home is a particular location within the spiritual dimension where that relationship is expressed. This does not mean that we cannot be within the physical body and still be exchanging that relationship with God. Should we be ready, we can begin to re-establish our original relationship with Him while still inhabiting this physical body.

This is why Moses, Jesus and all the saints have taught:

"'Love the Lord your God with all your heart and with all your soul and with all your mind.' This is the first and greatest commandment. And the second is like it: 'Love your neighbor as yourself.' All the Law and the Prophets hang on these two commandments." (Matthew 22:37-40, Jesus quoting Moses)

Fifth Principle: God has created a number of categories of living beings. The first are His Direct Expansions. The second are His Partial Expansions—those who have some individuality, but will never waiver in their relationship with Him. The third are the free souls. These living beings are individuals who have been given the complete freedom to love God or not. For these free souls (each of us), God sets up a continual testing process to give us the choice to stay with Him or not. This is the analogy of the "tree of life" from the Garden of Eden. God kindly asked Adam not to eat of the tree. Why was the tree even there? It was there because God was giving Adam the *choice* to obey Him or not.

Sixth Principle: While God domiciles within the spiritual dimension, He still pervades the physical dimension through His creative and communication features. God regularly sends messengers in the form of teachers to represent Him. The reason we do not "see" God within the physical world is because we do not want to see Him.

Seventh Principle: The physical world was set up for those who decide they want to enjoy life away from God. Here we can pretend to be independent, and try to accomplish our self-serving goals without God. This is symbolized in the analogy of Adam in Genesis:

> *The Lord God made garments of skin for Adam and his wife and clothed them. And the Lord God said, "The man has now become one of us, knowing good and evil. He must not be allowed to reach out his hand and take also from the tree of life and eat, and live forever." So the Lord God banished him from the Garden of Eden to work the ground from which he had been taken. After He drove the man out, He placed on (in front of) the east side of the Garden of Eden cherubim and a flaming sword flashing back and forth to guard the way to the tree of life.* (Genesis 3:21-24)

The *garments of skin* spoken of in Genesis are our temporary physical bodies. Because we decided to choose not to do God's will, desiring instead to become like Him (to *"become one of us, knowing good and evil"*). As a result, God banished us from the spiritual world (*the Garden of Eden*), and put up a border between the physical and the spiritual worlds (*cherubim and a flaming sword flashing back and forth to guard the way to the tree of life*).

The creation of the physical world might be compared to Dad building a young boy a treehouse in the backyard. The boy can now get away from the seeming control of the parents and feel that he is independent. In the treehouse, he feels that he is independent of his parents. The parents still keep a close watch on that treehouse, however. The boy never really is free from their control, however. But the treehouse gives him the illusion of independence.

In the same way, this physical universe is set up with the illusion that God isn't around. He is around, however. He is always there, watching and waiting patiently for us to reconsider our decision to abandon Him.

The treehouse analogy is a little weak because the treehouse is usually a simple box nailed into a tree with a ladder. The physical universe is designed with elaborate mechanisms that precisely reflect our consciousness and teach us along the way. At every step, we are given a physical body that matches our goals, desires and activities. Every activity in bodies of higher consciousness (i.e., human form) has a consequence. Just as parents often give their children who do bad (or even good) consequences to learn and grow from their actions, God sets up a consequential relationship between our activities and our future.

For example, child psychologists are now saying, after many years of research, that the best way of teaching a child is to set up reflective consequences for their actions. Say a child throws some food against the wall. As a consequence, the child will have to clean up the wall, clean up the room, and do chores to earn enough money to pay for the food that was wasted. This exercise, according to behavioral scientists, more thoroughly teaches the child than, for example, a spanking might.

Rather than it being a selective (prone to error) method as parents might apply in a consequential situation, God's physical universe is set up with an automatic mechanism of reflective consequences. In other words, He does not have to intervene and set up a consequence for us. Our bodies and physical environment are automatically programmed to do that, just as a video game might be programmed to respond to certain activities of its game players.

For example, let's say that we slugged someone at work. This sets up an immediate consequence for us to experience. Most likely, the immediate consequence is that we will precisely experience the pain we inflicted upon the other person when the other person slugs us back. Now should the other person not slug us back, we experience an array of other consequences as we get fired by the boss for our actions. Then we might have difficulty finding another job because we got fired for being violent at work. This might end up in us taking a construction job or other hard labor job—one that 'slugs us back' in different ways.

We discussed this before. In many instances, the full effect of our consequences will not be seen until the next lifetime. This is because sometimes this is the only way a precise consequence can be set up. For example, if we are wealthy, and we use that wealth to take advantage of poor people, then it would not be possible for us to experience the full effect of our actions without becoming poor. So we take on a physical body in a poor family or society during our next lifetime, and we are taken advantage by wealthier people. This gives us the full experience of how our activities affected others.

This reflective consequence mechanism of the physical world is perfect and completely fair. Many of those who question the existence of God ask the fundamental question: Why do some people suffer more than others? And why is there suffering in the world in the first place?

God created a perfect mechanism. It is perfect because God set it up with love in mind. Just as a parent has our ultimate benefit in mind when they issue consequential discipline, God is seeking our ultimate benefit with the design of the physical universe. God wants us to grow. He wants us to learn and reclaim that wisdom we once had before the fall. We must ultimately remember that these physical bodies are not *us*. They are temporary, virtual machines we drive around for a few decades. We get away unscathed (outside the wisdom we gain).

Why does God want us to gain wisdom? Because He wants us to enjoy the relationship we once had with Him. Like any of us, God is motivated by love. Because He loves us, He wants us to be happy. And He knows that returning to our relationship with Him will make us happy.

Consider the so many statements by God in Bible. Consider this statement by God speaking through Malachi:

> "But for you who revere my Name, the sun of right-eousness will rise with healing in its wings. And you will go out and leap like calves released from the stall."
> (Malachi 4:2)

Why is God's Name so important? To revere God's Name while in this physical world is to revere God. This is because, while a name of a physical body is different from the spiritual self, there is no difference between God and His Name. There is no duality within the spiritual world. The reference to God is non-different than Himself. This is why in multiple places in the Bible it is said:

"Blessed is he who comes in the Name of the LORD."

So Where is Hell?

Many religious philosophies discuss the possibility of going to hell. As a result, the fear and avoidance of hell is oftentimes the reason a person begins to attend a church, mosque or temple. A person threatened with eternal suffering in a hellish atmosphere will often react with fear and repentance.

It is taught that hell is a place of suffering: a place of anguish and unhappiness. It is taught that hell is a place where misery, sadness, pain, and suffering exist. Hell is said to be a place of heat and fire. Popular depictions of hell show people chained up in red-hot, fiery dungeons being tortured by monstrous horned devils. Anguish and pain are the most common features of this depiction.

This depiction assumes that we are not in hell right now.

But what about the pain, anguish, torture and emptiness existing here on this planet right now? What about the wars, the murders, the terrorists and the starvation around the world right now? What are these, then? What should we call the state of existence where millions of people around the world are dying of starvation? What should we call places that do not have clean water to drink and millions of people die from dysentery? What about places were people die from malaria? How about places where women are raped and murdered with little or no protection? What should we call the place where greedy bankers, CEOs and lawyers steal money from unsuspecting investors who put their trust in them? How about the place where hurricanes, earthquakes and tornados rip apart homes and lives? How about the place where oil gushes into the ocean and washes up upon the beaches, turning them black and poisonous?

What should we call the place where someone is locked up in a closet by lunatic parents and beaten or raped throughout their childhood? How about the place where someone is condemned as insane and locked up in a mental institution—tied down to their bed and given drugs that cause horrendous ghoulish nightmares? What shall we call the place where someone is jailed in a small cell as a criminal and subjected to violence and rape? What should we call the place where a person is locked in a dark cell and tortured as a political prisoner by a violent government regime?

Are these places not hellish? Are they not places of anguish and pain?

Surprisingly, most of us don't relate with these states as actually being hell. It would seem that these sufferings are not bad enough to be called hell. Possibly each of these instances did not occur in a hot-enough or fiery-enough place to be called hell. Perhaps because we don't see any horned people or fiery dungeons, we can't identify them as hell.

How about the rest of us, living more average lives here in our modern society?

Our sufferings begin at conception. Our bodies begin their lives by forming in a hostile environment—the womb. We find ourselves trapped inside this dark womb for many months. Research has revealed that not only do babies feel pain in the womb, but they are extremely sensitive. The slightest jolt creates a painful experience that can only be expressed by recoiling or trying to adjust. Microorganisms also live within the womb, irritating the baby's new skin.

When our bodies are finally pushed out of the womb we immediately cry because of the harshness of the new environment. We are born in pain, evidenced by our screaming. Of course, most of us do not remember this excruciating experience.

Throughout childhood, we must adapt to various harsh realities. Our bodies undergo various physical aches, pains, and diseases. These are often described by the expression, "growing pains." Feelings of intense hunger alternate with teething, bloating, gas, fever, nausea, mumps, measles, and other childhood maladies. A dose or two of laughter and a few games provide us with short breathers for respite.

Our dealings with others are also often painful as we grow up. Even innocent games can easily turn competitive and hostile. Children can be hurtful and callous towards one another. Seemingly innocent games like dodge ball hide the pain and mental anguish caused by other playmates, siblings and parents. Not many of us can say that we haven't been beaten up by another child or even our sibling as children.

We have little control during childhood. We are perpetually subjected to the whims of our parents, teachers and other adults—who may or may not have our welfare in mind.

Children do not cry by accident. We cry as children because we are either in some kind of pain, or feeling frustrated with our situation. Crying seems to do little to alleviate the pain and frustration we feel, however. It might bring us a little attention—which we crave—but this will not always be the type of attention we are looking for. We are not able to do much to change things, though we desperately try. We might win a few slight victories here and there as we throw a few tantrums. Many of us will learn to cry for affection as we strive to be loved. Our parents will often figure this means we want another toy or bottle of milk, however. After being given these things often enough, we also may start to think that perhaps this physical stuff is what we need to alleviate our pain and emptiness.

Once our bodies grow a little, we are thrust into school. This often feels more like prison. Our school experience results in new kinds of pain. Most of the other kids are as miserable as we are, and as a result, we struggle with each other, fighting for pecking order and attention. Our childhood soon becomes a race: Who can get others to like or even fear them the most. Many of us will simply struggle to fit in.

As our bodies grow older, we are introduced to new types of pain. Middle and high school opens an entirely new level of greed among our classmates. Sports and other activities, which bring attention to successful children, bring out stiff competition—often leading to violence and discrimination—as kids jostle for popularity.

As we age, new stresses are added: The pressure to get good grades, get into, pay for and get through a good college is added to the pressure of choosing a career. Getting through school usually means being forced to spend many hours each day memorizing mostly inconsequential facts and figures in order to pass exams.

Meanwhile, we experience so many heartaches, bouts of loneliness, growing pains, and the feeling of being trapped. Fights with parents can get worse, as our parents don't seem to understand us. Between the pressures of fitting in with our schoolmates and pleasing our parents, we find ourselves strung between two worlds, as we attempt to figure out our place in society. "What do you want to be when you grow up?" is the common question we're supposed to have an instant answer for.

These pressures lead to various mental and emotional anxieties. On top of this, we must deal with the issues of our parents. These may range from drug abuse and alcoholism to violence. Incest is a surprisingly frequent occurrence, especially among step-parents. Imagine being forced to live in a house with a rapist, and not being able to tell anyone for fear of their threats. Now why would this not be considered hell?

To add to these parental derangements, we will likely have to suffer from bullying, often from an older siblings. While schoolyard bullies can be devastating, having a bully in the next bedroom can be much worse. Again, under threat of worse punishment, we may be forced to keep quiet about these forms of suffering.

It is no wonder many teenagers in western society are on various drugs and medications. No wonder many are depressed and/or suicidal. No wonder many have developed perversions such as *self-mutilation*.

Childhood is full of pain. Childhood only appears attractive to reminiscing adults who have conveniently forgotten all the pain and suffering: A typical tendency of the mind.

As we graduate into adulthood, another level of suffering emerges. We now must figure out how to survive on our own in a competitive adult world. In the world of physical survival, there are so many people who make a living out of scamming or otherwise taking advantage of us. The free market system is set up to allow the bullies of society to con or otherwise take advantage of the weaker, nicer people.

In some places, we see wealthy corporations capitalizing on the efforts of children and poor adults to produce goods for wealthier people. Unbelievably, in some parts of the world, we also still see people being bought and sold as though they were commodities. Active slavery isn't as prevalent as it was just a century ago, but today there are still subtle forms of it in many societies. While wealthy people can make one million dollars during one phone call, others make a few cents or a few dollars per day toiling in drastic factory conditions, or laboring on industrial sized farms choked with pesticides. While some gorge themselves on super-sized meals, people in many parts of the third world are lucky if they can get a bowl of rice for the entire day. Oh, what a wonderful world we live in!

Regardless of where we live, and upon which economic level we stand, we experience an increasing level of discomfort and pain as our bodies age. None of us makes it through adulthood without becoming extremely sick on occasion. Most adult bodies get multiple colds and/or flu viruses each year. No one—not even those with the healthiest of bodies—is spared from a devastating and miserable illness at some point. This is why hospitals are constantly lined with sick people, suffering in pain and agony from either disease or injury.

Almost everyone ends up in the hospital at some point in their physical lives. There are thousands of different illnesses we can contract in our lifetimes. Medical books are thick with the various illnesses, and each sickness creates its own special form of misery.

Illnesses are directly related to our past or recent past activities, and there is little a physical body can do to avoid some of them. Escaping illness in our physical lifetime—though modern medicine tries heroically—is not possible. Quite simply, our physical body is designed to be inflicted.

In addition to the various pains associated with illness, there are many other stressors that affect us throughout our lives, causing us various degrees of discomfort and pain. There are so many environmental stressors our bodies must face. In many places, the seasons range from brutal cold, wet and snowy to boiling heat and sweltering humidity. Is there any place on the planet we are truly comfortable?

For this reason, many consider a tropical environment the perfect location. However even tropical places have their environmental problems: Mosquitoes, horrible rainy seasons (floods or hurricanes), and humid jungles that cause the body to sweat through the day and night are just a few of the many issues those tropical climates come with.

Add to this various human-created environmental problems including air pollution, water pollution, overcrowding, noise pollution and so many other stressors we've created within our modern society.

We face so many hassles from others, including people we work with. Our boss or management in general—or our peers—want to outmaneuver us as they gain authority over us.

Employees often wish they owned the company, but the business owners deal with their own range of stresses. These are associated with investors and stockholders, and the incredible financial challenges of staying in business. To this we add having to compete with other businesses that would just assume we were out of business.

There are so many other people-oriented stressors: Neighbors who disturb us. Disagreements or controversies between friends or family members. Crime and violence by those around us in one way or another. As soon as we think we have escaped one type of stress, another stressor arises. Just as we solve one challenge, a new challenge will present itself to take the first ones place.

In between so many of these pains and stresses are brief bursts of neural feedback that we consider pleasurable. But are these actually pleasurable? Actually, they are better described as relief than pleasure. These brief episodes of neurochemistry allow us to temporarily forget all the stresses and pains for a minute or two. For this reason, memory is often severely subjective.

A good example of this is the sexual orgasm. The orgasm is what many humans live for. Many strive for the sexual orgasm throughout their sexually active lives—continually seeking that momentary rush of neurochemistry. Humans will struggle for many years—enduring many hardships—to arrange their lives in such a way that will attract the opposite sex. Humans may even sacrifice their reputations and the health of their bodies to achieve this momentary urge.

Getting to the orgasm with a partner is not an easy task, however. First one must find a willing partner. This can get complicated, and can take months if not years of determined searching and dating. Through the process of finding a willing and suitable partner, we may endure painful confrontations; the pains of breakup; and many other forms of rejection. Then to get to the organism—assuming we have found a willing partner—we must partake in various forms of ritual: often referred to as foreplay. These rituals can take time, and if not done just so, the whole thing can be ruined. It is a tight-rope scenario. One slip-up—a bad joke, ill-timed flatulence, or a wrong move—could easily ruin the whole occasion, leading to embarrassment and pain. After all of this effort, the culmination—the orgasm—will only last for a few seconds, and sometimes may not happen at all. Then there is the disappointment of it coming too early.

Should the orgasm come, all the built-up expectations and anticipation will immediately be over—typically leaving let-down due to our expectation of fulfillment. For many this follows by a smoke or something to eat. Why so quick to move on to more consumption? Isn't the most sought after part of physical life satisfying? No. This is because the sexual organism is: 1) only fleeting; and 2) not satisfying to the transcendental inner self.

Often the sexual effort only leads to additional suffering. Should the man not perform well, he will be embarrassed and anxious, as his reputation becomes damaged. Should one of the partners have a sexual disease, they will both come to suffer from an often excruciating experience, which might bloom into AIDS, herpes or a number of other sexually-transmitted diseases.

Our attempts at other physical pleasures can be even more fleeting. The pleasures of eating good tasting foods, buying material goodies or other physical possessions offer brief flashes of neural feedback. A new car, house or other material item may be anticipated for many hours, days, or weeks in advance. They may also be accompanied by struggle and frustration to get them. They will usually require hard work, planning and dealing with people who want their own piece of the pie.

This is illustrated by the violence surrounding the dealing of drugs by international drug cartels. Each cartel struggles to dominate the distribution of their drugs, leading to bloodshed on each side.

Typically our plan for the acquisition is never what we envision. We think the new goodie will somehow fulfill us, but it never does. Once we get it, we are usually disappointed that it did not deliver any fulfillment. Once we get it, we are stuck having to take care of it and protect or maintain it. We have to work hard to reduce the potential that our acquisition may be stolen or otherwise damaged.

The ancient texts describe this in detail. They describe the three miseries attached to material acquisition: 1) The misery of obtaining the difficult-to-acquire possession; 2) The misery involved in protecting and maintaining the item; 3) And the misery associated with the loss or damage of the possession.

Most of us live our lives in perpetual fear. As children, we may be afraid of the bogeyman. Then we may be afraid of schoolyard bullies. Then we may be afraid of failing. Then we may be afraid of being embarrassed. Then we may be afraid of losing money. Then we may be afraid of getting sick or injured.

Then we may be afraid of being hurt by others. Then we may be afraid of dying. Fear drives so many of our actions and consciousness during our physical lifetimes.

Look carefully at the other organisms of this planet. Take a look at a bird—or any other animal for that matter. They are in a perpetual state of fear for their lives. This is evidenced by their quick motions of the head and their darting, watchful eyes. (Just try approaching them for a confirmation of this.) Most organisms deal with multiple threats from various organisms. Many are faced with terrifying situations: A bug is faced with monstrous creatures. Consider what a frog looks like to a fly: ferocious. Or what a cats with sharp teeth looks like to a mouse. Consider a rabbit faced with giant hawks, wolves, foxes and other beasts. Should they ambush the rabbit, they would devour it within minutes.

The human form faces similar frightening scenarios. These are caused by other animals, by other humans, by our environment and by our own technology. Machines, chemicals, weapons and bombs we have invented have become extremely dangerous. Millions of people die each year from automobile, plane, or train accidents. They move so fast that we are literally on the edge of death. The simplest intrusion—such as a deer in the road—can instantly cause a nightmarish and disfiguring accident if not death. Other threats we can thank our modern scientists for include various dangerous medications, genetic mutation, electromagnetic radiation, pesticides, toxic waste, air pollution and global warming. These modern threats more than replace any of the protective benefits of our technology.

The most brutal part of living in this physical environment is the loneliness. As we pretend to casually relate to our friends and relatives, underneath we are lonely. Why? We feel alone here in this physical world, where everyone is out for themselves. Those that seem to care tend to care sometimes and not care other times.

We feel alone when we discover that our friends are not real friends after all. We are lonely when we find out our friends are actually acquaintances out of convenience. When it is no longer convenient for them, we don't hear from them.

We feel alone when the family and relatives we depended upon for love go away or break up.

Just when we think we have adapted to this hostile physical environment, we are forcefully yanked away by death. Death rages in without notice to remove all of our attachments: our spouse, our friends, our family, our house, our car, our wealth or lack thereof—everything—is taken like a thief in the night.

Death creates a dread for every living organism. Death will snatch us away from everything. Some like to pretend to have joyous burials and wakes full of remembrance for the person who passed away. Beneath these masquerades are family members and friends who are in shock. They cannot believe that we are gone. They cannot believe that death is that close. This is because most of us feel that *we will never die*. Only others die.

So now we must ask again: How far away from hell is this? Does the constant state of alternating anxiety, illness, injury, sadness, anger, frustration, hate, loneliness, violence, and fear not qualify as hellish enough? Does the terrorism, torture, violence or starvation, hatred, prejudice and rape not qualify as hellish enough?

Or does the momentary fleeting absence of physical pain or brief neural surge qualify this world as being better than hell? And if it is above hell, how far above hell is it?

Sorry, but this is hell.

Yes, some of us live in a worse hell than others. Some of us—especially those living in lower forms of life—are living in a brutally more hellish hell than most of us. A living being subjected to a physical body designed for various levels of pain, old age, disease and death is in hell. The level of pain and suffering varies to species. The species in turn varies to consciousness.

Now what about that depiction of hell as a hot, fiery, burning place? We've all heard someone describe a particular pain as a "burning pain." We have also heard of situations where someone is "burning with anger," or "burning with desire." The 'burning fire' of material existence can range from these physical pains to the suffering related to the various fears of the world and the heated nature of selfish competition, violence and torture.

This is not to say that there are not other hellish planets worse than ours, to one degree or another. We can simply review the various species of life here on this planet to see just how variegated suffering can be among different life forms. Simply picking up a rock will reveal a tiny world of predators and violence among the insect world.

What? You don't believe that you could ever occupy a body of an insect? Think again.

The cause-and-effect mechanism within the physical world also explains the cycle of evolution and de-evolution. Yes, it is possible for a person to descend into the lower species of life. This is the very meaning of "going to hell." By living a life focused upon the animalistic activities of sex, violence, eating and defending without a meaningful search for God, the inner self during the human lifetime, we are subject to descending into the animal species by taking on a body *that most closely our consciousness and past activities at the time of death.*

Consider, for example, what species a person whose dog is the center of their lives will attain after this lifetime? Any guesses? Has anyone ever noticed how people begin looking like their dogs even during this lifetime?

This is critical, because we must understand that our actions and associations have consequences. We may not always realize the consequences of our actions in the immediate future. But we will indeed bring upon ourselves the consequences of our actions during our next lifetime if not during this lifetime.

This means that a person who engages in the needless torture or killing of innocent animals during their lives will likely suffer the exact punishment they inflicted upon others during the lifetime in which they had the choice: the human lifetime. If a person was responsible, for example, for killing 10,000 cattle during their career of cattle farming and meat-eating, the inner self will be committing themselves to at least 10,000 lifetimes within bodies of cows or other species to suffer the same gruesome death they inflicted upon those innocent cattle.

On the other hand, being less aggressive and more caring toward others will usually result in receiving less pain. This is the way the physical world has been designed, in order to educate us. There is a price for any selfish action. If we decide we want to try to control others for example — utilizing some sort of governorship or business ownership: this will require us to pay a stiff price for the opportunity and the results of such leadership. If we want to become comfortable at the expense of others, there will be a cost for that comfort.

This is the perfect design of the physical world. Everyone receives what they have dealt out when they had a choice. The human lifetime provides choice and intelligence not afforded by many other species. Therefore, how we utilize our human form is critical.

This also explains the age-old question of why some people are born into suffering in the world. Those who are born into suffering undoubtedly inflicted suffering upon others during their previous lifetimes. This is not to say that we should not be compassionate about others and try to help others. We should always have mercy upon others in less fortunate situations. But at the same time, we should not be blaming God or anyone else for the suffering of this world. The suffering of this world has been brought upon us by ourselves. We are the captains of our own ships, and collectively, members of the same ship.

Withdrawing from the world is only a temporary fix. Many propose that we need to transcend this painful world by withdrawing from our attachments. Many supposed spiritual practices teach we should meditate in an effort to withdraw from the sensory world — the goal being to merge into "nothingness" or "everything." However, methods that attempt to eliminate desire will not be successful. The living being is perpetually active, and must be attached to something (or stated more correctly, someone). The inner self cannot simply disconnect from desire.

This attempt to withdraw is no different than alcoholism or drug abuse in an effort to escape the pains of life. Suicide is also a form of withdrawal. None of these attempts to withdraw will result in any solution. As for suicides and lives spent inebriated, this simply results in taking on a ghost body for the duration of time that was cut short by the withdrawal. Our bodies have an intended lifespan depending upon our past activities (which can also be changed with activities of this lifetime). If we cut our physical lifespan short by committing suicide, drinking or drug-taking, we will live out the difference within our subtle ethereal body.

The ethereal or ghost body is particularly nightmarish because we are left in a state of being able to observe the physical events of the environment our gross physical bodies once lived within. But we cannot partake in those events. We cannot communicate with those we observe. We can only watch. This is particularly frustrating, because we cannot exchange relationships with those that we felt were close to us during our physical lives. This, however, is the perfect consequence of our behavior when we had a gross physical body — we wanted to withdraw.

Ghosts, by the way, are always looking to find ways back into the gross physical dimension. For this reason, they will frequently find alcoholics who regularly become drunk enough to drop their nervous system shields. As alcohol loosens (numbs) our grip on our body, this allows ghosts to temporarily gain control over the body. This is why we find that many alcoholics seem to become different people when they are drunk. It is because their bodies have become controlled by a ghost (sometimes even multiple ghosts) who take control over the body when they loosen their grip as they drink or take drugs.

Rather than try to withdraw and disconnect, the real solution is to become attached to the Supreme Person. This is our natural constitution, and the only way that we can permanently become detached from this hellish environment. Becoming attached to the Supreme Person solves a number of problems: Because He will protect and deliver us from suffering (and ghosts), we can depend upon Him. Because He is our Best Friend, we no longer need to experience the distress of loneliness. Because He is always there for us to console us, we do not have to be concerned with any future stresses of the physical world. Because He is from the transcendental world, with Him we can transcend our various physical miseries by focusing our senses, efforts, and results towards Him. By becoming attached to the Supreme Person, the various anxieties caused by being attached to these physical bodies will gradually evaporate.

The Perfect Love

We can know some qualities about who our true love is by the qualities we seek in them. They are caring. They are giving. They are kind. They are forgiving if we do something wrong. They never forget us even if we forget them. They are beautiful. They are ever-youthful (they don't get old and die on us). They are healthy and strong. They are funny. They are fun to be with. They share our most intimate details and keep our confidence. They understand us. They listen. They take care of us.

Who could this person be? How about we ask this differently: Who else but the Perfect Person could this be? Who else but the Person who owns and controls everything? Who else but the most beautiful person in the universe? Who else but the Eternal Supreme Person?

The central problem with our need for love is that it can only be satisfied by the Supreme Person. The reason why our lust is such a bottomless pit is because the source of this lust—love—only truly exists in connection with the unlimited Supreme Person. This is because the Supreme Person Himself is a limitless, bottomless lovable Person. Loving Him is an ever-deepening experience, which brings the living being complete joy and fulfillment.

Since the Supreme Person is the reservoir of true love, our ability to express and experience actual love is connected to our innate relationship with Him. If we are trying to enjoy without Him, or trying to be Him, we can hardly expect to connect with our natural ability to love. If we are trying to enjoy the world—attempting to consume it for our own satisfaction—we will not be able to relate with the Supreme Being. This is because the Supreme Person is a being of pure love—His love is pure and unconditional. His love is kind and tender. His love is forgiving and complete. Living beings in physical bodies pretending to love through relationships of exchange are simply not equipped to replace this deep, boundless source of love.

Most depictions of God are impersonal. People will refer to God as "love." Or they will refer to Him as "spirit." Some may even refer to Him as "everything," or worse, that we are all God. None of these depictions make logical sense. We are individuals, and we will remain individuals. We do not merge into each other. Love requires individuality, and each of us individually needs love. God is also an Individual. He is the Original Individual, and we are His offspring. Therefore, we become complete when resume our original relationship with Him.

Like a bull in a china shop, a selfish person cannot relate in the world of transcendental love. This is the reason we have these physical bodies: To play out our selfish desires in a place that is incompatible with the sensitive nature of the relationships that exist within the transcendental world.

Since we are not relating with Him and His world of love now, we cannot truly relate with other living beings with real love. When we are covered by selfishness, we see everyone in connection with what we can get from them. We are not able to see other living beings as they are, simply because we are covered by this cloud of lust. If, however, we become reconnected with the Supreme Person and are able to enter His world of love, our ability to see others as they truly are will allow us to truly love others.

When we speak of the ultimate love, we usually refer to a scenario where the lover gives 100% of themselves, without any conditions. Has this ever happened to us in this world? Have we ever met another human who didn't have any conditions upon the love that was given? If we have, we are extremely fortunate. With just about every human there are conditions for which love will be extended. For some it might be attractiveness. For others it might be family. For still others it might be age, or sexual preference. For still others it might be conditional on reciprocation, or at least acknowledgement. Would we be prepared to love someone who wanted to hurt us?

We can easily observe that the Supreme Being loves us unconditionally. How? Simply because He loves us even if we do not love Him back or even acknowledge Him. He loves us even though our activities are hurtful to Him. This is illustrated by the fact that we are away from Him now. Many of us in this physical world are ignoring Him now. Many of us who are not ignoring Him are trying to use Him to get something else. In either case, these kinds of actions would be considered hurtful to anyone who loved us.

He could easily force us to serve Him and pay attention to Him if He wanted. But this would not be love though, since love requires the freedom to love or not to love. Because the Supreme Person loves us unconditionally, He not only continues to love us despite our hurtful activities, but He has even given us a place where we can continue to ignore Him. Through all this, He is always ready to take us back when we are ready. Now that is true love.

Returning Home

The physical body is a temporary vehicle for the eternal spiritual inner self. Why are we so attached to this physical body? Why, despite the pain, disease, old age and other problems, are we so determined to insist that we are this body?

The reason we become so attached to the body is because each of us became determined, at some point, to be independent of God. We wanted to be free from God's presence and seeming domination. Rather than love and serve God, we wanted to be loved and served: We wanted what God has, in other worlds. This initial demand for freedom from God, and the desire to enjoy as God, created the incentive to be granted not only a physical body: but also a wall of false ego preventing us from seeing God and realizing that we are not God.

This wall of false ego is strong. It pervades the mind at every step. Every function of the mind comes with the assumption that we are the body and there is nothing else to existence. Even though from a logical and scientific basis (as we've shown here) this doesn't make sense, our mind persuasively guides us towards conclusions that we are the all and all, and nothing else is as important as we were. This gives us the constant illusion that we are the body and God does not exist. Even though our physical eyes are obviously limited in scope and bandwidth—we assume that unless we see it with our eyes, it must not exist. This of course is not a scientific conclusion, yet this is the conclusion that scientists continually assume in their research.

The reason we wanted to be separate from the Supreme Being is because we became envious of Him. We wanted to have what He has. This is a common development among those who are given freedom.

Due to this enviousness—combined with our constitutional need to be attached to something—we became attached to the temporary physical body and the temporary physical world. The result is our attempt to enjoy an existence away from the Supreme Person.

The physical body is simply a tool designed for that purpose. It is the vehicle we use to attempt to set up a virtual universe where we could play lord while others respect and serve us.

It doesn't work out so well. While we are able to get some goodies, and we think we are getting respect from others, the world also takes these away. The physical world is designed to teach us. It is designed to reflect ourselves back at us: Like a grand mirror, all of our greed, lust and selfishness are reflected right back with our placement into certain types of bodies and circumstances.

It is not hard to see that without the selfish activities of its inhabitants, this physical environment could be a lot more inhabitable. If the living beings who occupied other bodies were kinder and more giving, many of the hells of the planet would not exist. But then again, if we weren't so selfish and greedy, we wouldn't be here in the first place.

The deep-seated sense of joy we feel when we help or care for others indicates that our natural identity is tied to loving service rather than selfish behavior. It is not a coincidence that loving service helps relieve the suffering of others. What we probably don't see is that loving service also relieves our own suffering. Research has found this proclivity among those who suffer from depression or post-traumatic stress syndrome: They find relief when they go out and help others.

The fact that loving service benefits us reveals that our natural constitution is related to being a servant and a giver than a self-centered, greedy enjoyer.

We are often shocked at finding out that some third world regime is causing the suffering of its own citizens. We wince when we discover that a fellow human has tortured another, or has blown up a building with innocent people inside. These things are shocking to us, but those people who did those horrors do not share our opinion. They do not look much different than we do. They eat and sleep just as we do. They feel justified for their acts. Unbelievably, they feel they have a valid reason to cause the suffering of others.

Research on criminals has discovered that the overwhelming majority of criminals feel somehow justified in their crimes. They felt they were somehow forced to commit suffering upon other humans. Why is this? Are these people evil while we are not? Are we completely innocent of ever causing the suffering of another, even unintentionally? Quite simply, progressive selfishness causes increased insensitivity to others, maturing to a point where ones selfish concerns outweigh the suffering of others.

The world we live in is a reflection of our activities and our consciousness. Our original enviousness of our Best Friend is the cause for our initial fall into this hellish physical world. The root feeding this hellish tree is our desire to enjoy as the Supreme Being enjoys. This act of 'eating the fruit' of this tree of envy is *the original sin*.

The physical world was designed to enable us to recover from this disease of envy. It was designed perfectly to allow us to grow and learn that selfishness and enviousness do not make us happy. This world is designed to teach us that only love will satisfy us. When we sow love, we receive love. When we sow hatred, we receive hatred. These reactions should illustrate to us the preferable consciousness.

Should we decide to exchange our enviousness for a re-newed relationship of loving service with the Supreme Person, we would be starting our journey home. Our body and mind would be transformed from frustrating tools for enjoyment into vehicles able to help return us back to our original relationship with God.

Should we decide to return home, our lives would become surcharged with a renewed purpose and direction. Suddenly, life makes sense to us. Suddenly, we have a reason for existing.

Then, at the end of this lifetime, or perhaps at the end of the next, we will return home. We will re-enter the world we intui-tively belong: A place where everyone cares for each other. A place where we engage in fun, loving relationships. A place where we always have a real Best Friend and Companion.

God is, after all, a Person. He has a personality, a will and a propensity for love. He is not a vague force floating in the sky.

So how do we get started on our return home?

Let's say that you have a son who, as soon as he turns 18, turns to you and says, *"I don't want to be here. I want to leave. I don't want you telling me what to do anymore. I want to have my own house and my own job. I don't like you anymore. I want my freedom!"* As he yells this, he storms around your house, breaking things and punching walls.

What do you do? Certainly, you are hurt by such statements. After all the love and care you've had for him over the years, you are saddened that he does not care to be with you. After all the things you have done to keep him safe. You have fed him, changed his diapers, and potty trained him. You played ball with him and read him bedtime stories. Now he just wants his freedom. Now he says he hates you.

Because you love him, you send him off to get his freedom. You give him a car and make sure he has enough money to find a new place to live, and enough to hold him over until he gets a job. You tell him you hope he goes to college and you offer to pay. You tell him if he ever needs help he can always call you.

Then you say goodbye. Your son hurriedly packs his bags and takes off in the car, and flips you off as he drives away.

Two years later, he calls you for the first time. Of course, you take the call. Though you are still hurting from his exit and from the fact that he's never called you, you have been missing him and you are happy to hear from him. You are certainly hurt that he hasn't been in touch, but you are also forgiving. He is, after all, your son. And you still love him.

Now he is calling because he wants to come back to your house and live with you again. He wants to stay at home and go to college. He wants to be a family again. He wants to forget the past and just come home.

It's not so easy, however. Things have changed. What he did two years earlier really hurt you. You also do not know if he is ready to come back to live with his parents again. Is he prepared to be a contributing member of the household? Or will he pull the same stunt as he did before? Is he just trying to take advantage of you to get some free rent? Or is he being honest when he says he just wants to be with you again?

As these questions loom, it appears to you that the wise thing to do is to spend a little time with the young man to get reacquainted. Perhaps you invite him out for lunch first, and then maybe dinner at the house. During this time, you are checking and testing a few things. Perhaps you ask him to do a thing or two for you, and you are interested to see how well he does those. In other words, he has to prove to you that he is sincere and really ready to come home.

Over a month or two, you gradually get to know each other again, and you feel convinced that he has changed over these two years. The world has taught him some important lessons. After some time, you are ready to take him back and give it another go, because you see that he is sincere.

This is not so far from the situation that has occurred between us and our Best Friend, God. For eons (there is no time in the spiritual world) we were with God, enjoying a loving relationship with Him. He was our life and soul. We served Him with great joy and He also did many things for us. He cared for us greatly. But He also gave us the free will to love Him or not.

At some point we wanted to go. We rejected God. We wanted to enjoy like Him and we wanted our freedom. Because we can never really be away from God (as His presence is pervasive) He set up a virtual world where for all tense and purposes, we feel free of Him. At the same time, because He cares for us, He also sets up a mechanism to help us learn and grow while we are away.

Now what if we suddenly say we want to come back and be with Him. Will He just take us back, no questions asked? He has been hurt by us, and now He needs to know that this is not just a whim: Are we serious about coming back to Him? Are we ready to come back to Him and live within the spiritual environment (where there is no envy or hatred, only play, love and service). In other words, we cannot come back to Him while we are still envious of Him and others. This just will not work. We simply are not ready yet.

So what happens? God does not just turn us away. Rather, He submits us to a process of learning that *prepares* us for returning to Him and the spiritual world. Some of the process tests our desire: How badly do we want to return? Some of the process tests our resolve: Are we ready to give up certain things to return to Him? Some of the process tests our persistence: Do we still want to return to Him after many trials and tribulations? Some of the process re-acquaints us to the environment of the spiritual world: how to be kind and forgiving to others. In all, this process is exhaustive, and it is personal. It tests us and prepares us specifically.

We do not always pass the tests. But whether we pass or not, they make us stronger. They also weed out those who were just wanting to go to heaven because they heard that heaven was a cool place. They weed out those who are just pretending to be religious to impress others. They weed out the non-serious people from those who seriously and sincerely want to be with God again.

In other words, are we saying we want to return to God just to get out of a rough situation? Do we just want to be "saved" from having to suffer the consequences of our selfish activities? Or do we truly want to re-establish our relationship with God?

For the Skeptics

Even though the understanding of the physical world and the transcendental world outlined here logically fits with all of our scientific observations, there are still many skeptics—especially with regard to the existence of the Supreme Being. In fact, most of us have been skeptics at one point or another, and skepticism can be a good thing, because only through skepticism can we resolve the real questions about our identity. In fact, today many people are skeptical of the teachings of the major organized religions because many of the world's scriptures simply do not fit with scientific observation. This is because these teachers are presenting their philosophies without a true understanding of what those scriptures and those earlier saints actually taught.

The fundamental problem of most organized religions today is that their teachers have been appointed through political processes. Their focus therefore is to give deference to the political agendas of previous church or temple administrations rather than be focused on the intentions and lessons of God.

This has resulted in stubborn and arcane interpretations of scripture that do not respond to the realities of the physical world. They do not fit with scientific observation because they have not being presented by living saints on behalf of the living God. This is because those teachers are beholden to the committees and the political associations of their organized religions, rather than beholden to the living God.

In other words, they do not enjoy a loving relationship with God: They enjoy political relationships with church and temple administrators, and councils of cardinals, deacons and other political committees of men and women.

As one compares these arcane interpretations of scripture by religious organization teachers to modern scientific texts, many feel the scientific texts present a more practical approach to the universe because the scientific approach tends to more closely match observation. This is primarily because of modern science's advantages from the perspective of the conversation. Atheistic modern scientists currently dominate the conversation with most of the media outlets, driven by a secular culture that has a desire to separate faith from science. This has isolated those who are scientists and believers. A scientist with faith is typically blacklisted from scientific journals and the conversation with the media. This gives the atheistic scientific theories an unfair advantage in the debate.

This does not necessarily mean that modern atheistic science is offering a more scientific conclusion for the creation of the universe, however. Their theories propose a scenario where the universe randomly appeared from a massive accidental explosion. They propose that life, personality and the existence of love was the result of some random atoms coming together to create highly organized complexity. They propose that the highly functional earth, cells, DNA, sun, atom and solar system occurred accidentally from one random nuclear explosion eons ago.

Not only are these scenarios illogical, but they are unscientific because there is virtually no evidence to back them up. They are quite simply, theoretical speculations with absolutely no proof or logic. How could life come from no life? How could an explosion producing the universe come from nothing? And where did the original nuclear forces come from that started the big bang explosion? How could these original forces create the organized structures of the universe without an organizing force? And how could love, personality, emotion and the innate feeling that we are eternal come from an accidental (and unlikely, according to even the most staunch big bang theorists) combination of chemicals?

This theory of the universe would be in direct contradiction to the first law of thermodynamics: The first law says that energy must be conserved: It can be transformed from one state to another, but cannot be created or destroyed. Where then, did the tremendous energy come from that created the gigantic universe we see around us? Could this have come from the energy residing within one singular point of nothingness, as the big bang theorists propose?

One of the problems with this theory is that at some point, random chemicals had to form life. Furthermore, that original life had to have the desire to survive: according to Darwin's theory of evolution, 'survival of the fittest' required an innate desire to survive. This desire to survive means that a group of chemicals somehow began to differentiate themselves from "dead" chemicals. After all, why desire to survive if there is no basic difference between a "living" batch of chemicals and a "dead" batch of chemicals? Noting the difficulty of survival among the dangers of the elements, it would seem that being "dead chemicals" would be the path of least resistance—the far easier path— for a batch of chemicals. Why would these original "living chemicals" suddenly desire the difficulty of survival? And how could they differentiate themselves from the "dead chemicals" if there was no "being" to observe the difference between "dead chemicals" and their own "living chemical" structure?

Quite simply, there is no logical reason why dead chemicals would accidentally group together, and then begin desiring to survive as living chemicals. What would be the impetus for such a new desire?

Furthermore, this theory cannot logically explain the existence or creation of personality, love and the self-existence of the individual. Again, they propose that these characteristics accidentally arose from random chemical reactions.

By far the most scientific approach was proposed by the Greek philosophers such as Plato and Socrates, who proved logically that living matter must come from life, and there must be an organizing force from which the creation of the universe stemmed. This means, they concluded, that there must be a permanent nonphysical universe that houses that organizing force. They also suggested that this nonphysical force must also have, at the very least, the potentials of what was created in the physical universe.

This means that the nonphysical creative force must contain at least the individual elements existing here: Personality, love, compassion, desires, and all the energy to produce the electromagnetics that compose physical matter.

Therefore, since we are each individuals, this nonphysical force must also contain individuality. This means that this nonphysical force must be an individual: a person, with personality, emotions, desires and so on. We are now describing God.

So why are western scientists so bent on not accepting the existence of God? From a secular view, they are slanting away from religious faith because they see the acceptance of a Supreme Being as unempirical. They claim that faith is something that cannot be proven. Theories such as the big bang also require faith. They are not only grossly unempirical: they also contradict the laws of nature. Yet today's scientific community purposely stays away from topics of faith because individual scientists do not want to lose credibility among their peers (and those who delve into these topics do lose credibility). This is not unlike the situation occurring amongst many organized religions.

This mutual position by both sides has created the pseudo-rift between science and the existence of a Supreme Being.

This rift is only a development of the past four or five decades, however. A majority of the greatest scientists of the past five centuries (and practically every scientist previous) declared that they were men of faith, or in some sense accepted the existence of a Supreme Being. These include Einstein, Bell, DiVinci, Mendeleev and so many others. Practically every western scientist through the mid twentieth century was a person of faith. It was only after the 1960s did we start to see so many scientists opposed to faith in God. Dr. Einstein commented:

"I want to know how God created this world. I am not interested in this or that phenomenon, in the spectrum of this or that element. I want to know His thoughts. The rest are details."
(*The Expanded Quotable Einstein*, Princeton University Press, 2000 p.202)

So the skeptics must now ask ourselves why we are so opposed to the existence of a Source of life. Every single cosmologist accepts that the universe has a source. No scientist believes that the universe simply existed forever. The evidence of matter moving outward (called the Hubble constant, discovered a few decades back by cosmologists Hubble and Ho) points to a single creation point. The universe didn't appear from out of nowhere. Why should we be insistent that the point of creation did not come from a Supreme Being? Such a theory would be no less scientific than the theory that the universe came from a random grouping of nuclear forces (that came from where?). Furthermore, where did the energy come from that produced personalities, love, and individuality?

Okay, so let's say you are still not convinced. Let's say that even with the tremendous evidence of an individual Creator, you do not believe that God exists. You now fall into the category known as an "agnostic." Now let's realistically consider your current options as you prepare for death:

Option One: Insist—though there is no evidence for it—that the universe was created by a random, accidental explosion, and God does not exist. You must now assume that love is simply a cruel development of accidental evolution and is simply an error of the instinct of survival. (So why love family or spouse?) You must also insist that all of the visions, realizations, reveries and miracles that have been documented in our spiritual texts and among the thousands of near death experiences were either hallucinations or urban legends. By necessity, you also must accept that you will not survive after death. You will simply cease existing, and dissolve into nothingness, even though you have maintained your existence throughout a changing physical body during this body's lifetime.

Option Two: You trust that life had to come from life. You assume that the living portion of every organism came from a Living Source, and this Source comes from a dimension transcendental to the physical dimension. You trust that love is real, and love is our highest aim because each of us was created by a Loving Person who cares for each of us. You accept that we are all searching for that perfect person because we are away from God.

Let's now consider these options. From a purely logical, scientific and *risk-versus-reward* scenario, which option would be preferable? Consider first the risk of taking Option Two that God exists. What is the loss of such an option? What is the downside? If we trust that God exists and He doesn't, where does that leave us? Are we in any way disadvantaged if there is no life after death? Is there any risk in believing there is no spiritual world if there isn't? Is there any risk in having faith in a Personality in the form of God that we can turn to?

Let's consider, on the other hand, the risk of Option One. By insisting on Option One we must deny God's existence. What is the risk of this? If God *does* exist, and we are wrong, then where does that leave us? If we choose not to take any course of action to grow spiritually, then where are we if the spiritual world does exist? If we refuse to trust in God and God exists, then what?

God will be greatly offended. God's representatives and loving servants will also be offended. Everyone dwelling amongst God from the spiritual dimension will be offended. In this condition, we will be turned away from the possibility of entering the spiritual world for a very long time. Taking this option will deny us any opportunity to use this human form to return home, and it could take millions of lifetimes to once again have the opportunity to inhabit a human form.

Not having a trust in God will also leave us with an existence filled with only the physical pains and fleeting pleasures of a temporary physical body and mind. We will be focused upon the animalistic pleasures that come with this physical body. This will lead towards animal tendencies. This will likely lead us to take on the body of an animal. In the animal body, we won't have to think about God. We won't have to avoid people who believe in God because we will be amongst our own kind: Other living beings that are ignorant of God. We will simply suffer the violence and the pains (with fleeting pleasures) of the lower species, as we transmigrate from one body to the next in an empty world of loneliness—surrounded only by temporary family members.

We risk this possible existence simply because we chose to insist that God doesn't exist, when actually, we really didn't know. We simply selected door number one instead of door number two.

Have you ever purchased insurance? Why? If you didn't know whether there would be an accident or not, why did you err on the side of the possibility that there would be an accident and spend the money to purchase insurance? In this decision, the likelihood of an accident is extremely low. It may be on the order of one out of a million or more that you would need the insurance. Yet you bought the insurance anyway.

What are the odds of God's existence to the skeptic? Let's just say for the skeptics' sake it is 50/50. If you had a 50/50 chance of a catastrophic accident would you not buy the insurance?

Certainly, any reasonable person preparing for death would at least take out an insurance policy on God's existence. What do we have to lose?

Chapter Five

The Pain of Death

The blunt reality is that pain accompanies death in most instances. There is a good reason for this, however. A very good reason. When we come to understand why we have pain as we are dying, we will begin to appreciate pain. This appreciation will in turn help us to deal with the pain.

First let's discuss what pain is. Then we'll get to why pain is so important.

Most of us live our lives trying to avoid pain. Many even grade happiness on how little pain our bodies have. Here we have provided the evidence showing that the body is merely a temporary vehicle for an inner self. As a result, we can know that pain is also temporary. We also know by experience that we each feel pain virtually throughout our physical lives to different degrees. What is pain and how can we live with it?

The Anatomy of Pain

On a strictly physical basis, pain is transmitted through the nervous system from nerve endings called *nociceptors*. Nociceptors are located around the body, amongst just about every tissue system and organ system. The nociceptor is an electromagnetic waveform receptor. It has a designated threshold of waveform reception, beyond which it stimulates a waveform response. This is an alarm of sorts. The alarm travels through the nerve channels to the brain. The mind assembles a holographic map of the body, and this holographic mapping indicates the location of the nociceptor alarm. The specifications of this alarm are reflected onto the mindscreen to be viewed by the inner self. Sometimes the reflection of the pain signal will not exactly locate the pain signal's precise origin—stimulating an approximation of the location. This is called *referred pain.*

Pain has many classifications. It can be acute, chronic, referred, inflammatory, or even phantom. Phantom pain occurs when the pain appears to be coming from a part of the body that was amputated or otherwise lost. This alone indicates a subtle, energetic signaling system going on here. Pain is not as simple as we would like it to be.

There are several messages inherent within the design of pain. First and most obvious, pain is nature's way of telling us we need to solve a physical problem. We need to address something that has gone wrong in the body. The solution is most easily related to removing the cause. Sometimes, however, it is too late in the process. The damage has been done. Removing the cause may not remove the pain. This type of pain is caused by inflammation. The damage has stimulated a healing response, and the body is attempting to repair the damage by sending in blood, lymph, macrophages, neutrophils, plasmin and fibrin— likely a combination thereof. If the cause is removed, inflammatory pain will usually subside once the repair process has made substantial progress.

Incidentally, nature can assist in this process of repair with inflammation-reducing herbs such as goldenseal, garlic, cayenne, basil, willow, ginseng, turmeric, guggul and others.

If the original cause is not removed, the inflammation may become chronic. Chronic inflammation is the cause of most degenerative and autoimmune disorders. The body is constantly trying to repair damage created by recurring agents. This might be toxic chemicals, poor dietary habits, or other environmental inputs. As long as this input continues, the body's tissues will continue to be damaged. The inflammation and the pain associated with it will thus continue.

In some cases, chronic inflammation may be caused by an infectious agent. Here the infection is the cause. Since the immune system is unable to remove it, the damage it creates causes ongoing inflammation.

Then there is the natural degeneration of the body that comes with age. Degeneration from age can also cause inflammation. As even a healthy body ages, inflammation will gradually outpace the body's ability to repair the damage. This kind of inflammation will inevitably cause some chronic pain. It is often the result of a lifetime of wear and tear. It is thus unavoidable to some degree.

Chronic inflammation and pain can be substantially ameliorated with a diet of whole, plant-based foods, plenty of pure water, exercise, fresh air and sunshine. This will help decrease the burdens of poor input on our immune system, and speed up the repair process. As the repair process continues, the frequency and intensity of inflammatory pain can be decreased.

At the same time, we might be able to reduce the frequency and intensity of inflammation with other strategies. But in the end, pain is unavoidable. Just as a car is built with gauges that feed back oil, gas and heat levels, the body is designed to feed back pain sensations. Like the gauges, pain provides a clear indication of the condition of the body. It also reveals the existence of the viewer of the pain: the inner self.

Tolerating Pain

This means that every one of us, at some point in our lives, must learn to tolerate pain. We must learn to deal with it. We simply cannot make it through a lifetime of the physical body without dealing with its pain. The body was built to receive pain. It was built to receive a little pleasure as well. This creates a balance between the pains and pleasures of our bodies. Most of us have experienced many of the pleasures related to the body during the early and middle stages of the body. During our body's youth and middle ages, our bodies were fitter and more capable of fighting off diseases and healing injuries. This gave the body more opportunity to receive the body's pleasurable responses, driven by neurotransmitter feedback such as dopamine and serotonin.

During the last stages of the body's lifetime, the body's design makes it more vulnerable to chronic pain and inflammation. The healing response is slower, and the cells' ability to produce dopamine is reduced. This leaves us with a body with a greater likelihood of pain and less potential for pleasure.

What this all means is that we must gradually learn to tolerate the additional pain and the reduced pleasure. It doesn't mean that we give up all the strategies to reduce pain, however. We can still do all the things mentioned above, that will reduce our body's pains. We can also include herbs that tend to calm and soothe the pain response. These include hops, skullcap, basil, lavender, sage and St. John's wort.

While these can help, the solution to greater pain is to rise above it and reach for spiritual life. This is the actual purpose for pain—one that brings about a condition of pain tolerance. Let's review the science behind pain tolerance a bit further.

Some people are very tolerant and can withstand lots of it. Boxers, rugby players, football players, long distance runners, swimmers and other sports persons can tolerate excruciating pain as they train for and compete in contests. Others, on the other hand, might run or swim a lap and give up.

Dentists and anesthesiologists understand that there is a huge range of pain tolerance between people. At the dentist's office, some people do not even need Novocain. Others want to be knocked out with nitrous oxide. Some people cannot tolerate even the faintest pain sensations. They exert great effort to avoid it. Others will approach life head on—colliding with painful experiences on their way towards accomplishing their goals. This variance in pain tolerance is because we all have relative degrees of *pain sensitivity* with our bodies.

Indeed, many cultures have varying acceptable notions of pain. Some cultures undertake such traditions as fire walking and body piercing. Other cultures pamper their bodies with air conditioning and hot baths; whimpering with the slightest of temperature deviation. Soldiers have been known to endure extreme pain, while their leaders are often sensitive to the slightest of discomforts or challenges.

We also can also see huge variances between tolerances for suffering among different societies around the world. Some countries consider a small percentage of the population being homeless and cold as great suffering. Other societies deal with massive starvation, dehydration, and even mass genocide. Although none of these situations is acceptable in a world where some live in excess, it is easy to see a range of tolerance when it comes to human suffering around the world.

Why such a vast difference in tolerance to pain and suffering? If we were simply chemical machines, and pain was strictly a biological response, we would each respond the same to the same amount of pain. Yet this is not reality. Such a variance in pain sensitivity can only indicate that some of us—through training, conditioning or otherwise—feel more *connected* or *attached* to our body than do others.

This can be illustrated by measuring physical consciousness and pain tolerance together. It is widely accepted amongst anesthesiologists that the less conscious a person is, the less sensitive they will be to pain. This is why invasive surgical anesthesia will usually consist of giving a sedative and anesthetic concurrently. This puts the person into a state of unconsciousness: they lose their awareness of the body. There are exceptions, however. Sometimes a person may be sedated and still be aware. This rare problem is called *anesthesia awareness.*

Physical consciousness is the level of focus we might have upon our physical body at any point in time. After all, we must be conscious of something in order to be connected to it or attached to it. This attachment to our body is thus the key element associated with pain sensitivity and tolerance.

If we accept that each of us is the inner self and not the physical body, then we must accept that the pain and suffering our body experiences is not actually happening to *me*. If the pain is not happening to the self, the only way we will dread it and suffer from it is due to a misidentification with the body and an attachment to the body.

Let's use an analogy: Imagine that we bought a new car that we really liked. As we started driving it around, we began identifying ourselves with it. Say it is a sports car. We will feel that we are 'sporty' and cool when we drive this car. As this identification grows, we gradually become attached to the car. As we become increasingly attached to it, we become increasingly sensitive about any scratch or dent it might receive. If someone were to scratch our brand new car, or knock into it while parking, we might become very upset, even though we did not directly feel the scratch or bump. Why do we get upset even though we don't feel it? Because we are attached to the car and identify with it. We have been focusing more closely upon the car and its value to us. This focus increases our attachment and identification with the car.

What if instead, we bought an older car with plenty of dents and scratches. Consider it also had an ugly color and was not a very "cool" car. Would we identify as much with the car? Would we have the same attachment to the car? No. We would likely just consider the car good transportation. We would get in it, drive it, and then get out of it as fast as possible. We would not be so proud of it. If someone scratched it or knocked it while parking we'd not be very bothered. Another scratch or dent would not make much of a difference to us.

Let's consider that the *same* scratch or dent was put into each of the cars, under the conditions mentioned above. The *same* scratch or dent would affect us substantially differently.

We can conclude that the attachment and identification with our body reduces our pain tolerance. Greater attachment and identification with the body brings about a greater focus and physical consciousness upon our body. This is sometimes referred to as greater pain sensitivity. The more we are conscious of the body, the more pain sensitivity we will have. This is the central theme in surgical anesthesia, as the reduction of consciousness is the critical element.

This means that we can increase our pain tolerance by taking our focus away from the body. Instead of being focused on every little pain of the body and what this pain means to our body's future, our attention can be put elsewhere.

We can see this effect immediately in children. When a child is playing outside with friends, they will often be oblivious to a scrape on the knee, for example. Mom might really be focused on the injury, but the child may just keep playing. This is because the child's intentions and focus are on playing the game and not on the body.

Along with identification and attachment, the intentions we hold for the physical body are key considerations for pain sensitivity. Our various plans and expectations to utilize our body to achieve future pleasure will naturally result in a greater concern about anything that might endanger those plans. For example, losing our eyesight would not be so conducive to our future expectations of seeing the world around us. This makes us extra sensitive about our eyes.

In the same way, if we had plans to drive our car across the country, we would be very concerned about how the car was running prior to the trip. Any potential engine problem will be met with increased focus and concern because of the long drive.

Physical pain by itself is merely a signal that our body may be in danger. We can respond to each pain as a signal and act upon it; or we can dwell on each and every painful throb, dreading the thought of the pain continuing into the future, where it might disrupt our hopes and dreams for the future.

An example of the relationship between intention and pain sensitivity is an athlete who will endure tremendous pain for the sake of winning a race. A competitive long distance runner will run hundreds of miles per week for many years for the sake of winning that one big race. During their training, the runner may bring upon the body an almost unbearable amount of pain: The kind of pain we could easily compare to being held within a torture chamber. Yet the runner, because he or she is attached to the goal rather than the body's comfort, will endure that pain as a mere byproduct of preparing for the contest. Their attachment to the body's comfort is thus minimized by the purpose of the training. They intend to win, or at least perform well in the race.

On the other hand, a competitive runner determined to avoid pain would not do so well in the big race or during the training runs. As soon as any pain or discomfort arises, the runner will slow down or stop to avoid the pain. The winning runner accepts pain as part of the run and does not focus on it. The slower runner is focused upon avoiding the pain. This is due to the slower runner being less attached to winning and more attached to the body's comfort.

It is not as if the losing runner did not want to win. And in many cases, the losing runner may have longer legs and an otherwise better capability to run faster. The losing runner simply did not want to win as much as the winning runner did.

The winning runner's body will certainly feed back more pain signals, however. But since the winner has a greater focus upon winning the race, the pain didn't matter as much.

Another example of the relative effect of pain is self-mutilation. Today there are millions of kids inflicting their own bodies with razors, knives, pins and other painful tools. Surveys on self-mutilation reveal that kids do this in response to their feelings of frustration with the world around them. They feel empty and hopeless. Many describe having a feeling of numbness. Through self-mutilation, they say they hope to achieve a connection to reality.

In reviewing many of these cases, researchers have discovered that kids do not feel much pain when they self-inflict. They are more focused on filling their emptiness than on their bodily pain at that moment. Proving this point, many of these same kids have stated that they *do* feel great pain when involved in an accidental injury. They experience normal pain sensitivity when they are focused on their bodies' pleasure. On the other hand, when they are focused on seeking some kind of fulfillment ("filling the hole") from self-mutilation, they don't feel the pain.

Self-mutilation is surely an absurdity to most. For most of us, it is difficult to understand why someone would willingly inflict pain upon himself or herself. Some feel the same about certain athletes and sports, as we've discussed. Some would feel that these people are a bit insane to inflict this kind of pain upon their bodies for the purpose of winning a couple of contests.

In fact, in many of today's long distance races, there are tens of thousands of runners. There is little or no chance of most of these runners finishing first. In some marathons there can be as many as 100,000 runners, most of which will finish an hour or more behind the winner. They have no chance of winning. Why do they run the race, then? Why do they run 26 excruciating miles and bring this sort of pain upon themselves? Is this not much different than self-mutilation?

Athletes and self-mutilators are not much different. They are both simply focused upon achieving a particular objective, which at that moment outweighs the importance of comfort. Their attachment to the intended result overrides the pain.

And what are they both focused on? Fulfillment. They are each seeking fulfillment. The slow marathon runner who knows he or she will finish 75,000th or worse feels that by completing the race, they will somehow become fulfilled in some other way other than winning. Just completing the race might fill the empty hole. In some cases, attention from their family members or work associates might play a role as well.

This type of detachment also explains how prisoners-of-war can tolerate extreme conditions of torture and survive. During their torture, they are forced to detach from the pain as they try to focus upon other things. As a result, prisoners often pray and in general become focused on their spirituality. This detaches them from their horrible physical circumstances.

If we look at areas of the world that are poor and suffering we see the same thing. We see that people who are suffering tend to put more focus upon God. This detaches them from their suffering. For example, in a study done at the International Center for Health and Society at the University College London (Nicholson *et al.* 2009), 18,328 men and 21,373 women from 22 countries in Europe were surveyed. Those who attended religious services were significantly less likely to describe their health as being poor. This relationship was even stronger among people with chronic and longstanding illnesses in the study.

Because these people had put more focus on their spiritual lives, they became more tolerant of their suffering. Because chronic illnesses are most likely to be accompanied by pain, we can see that this directly correlates with pain.

We can see the relativity of pain sensitivity elsewhere in our lives. For example, the more attached we are to a particular event or person, the more something affecting that event or person might cause us pain, trauma or frustration. We can see this when people become wrapped up in sporting events—becoming attached to particular teams. In sporting team attachment, a team loss can significantly disappoint those attached to that team's results. For those who are not so attached to that team or sport, the loss would not affect them emotionally. For those unattached to a team, they have little emotional reaction to one result or another.

Becoming attached to another person can also become a source of pain. The more attached we become to that person, the more their death or breakup will cause us pain. The bottom line is that the level of pain we experience in any event is always relative to the amount of attachment we have.

This assures us that physical pain is relative to our attachment to our body and the specific intentions we have for our body. Physical pain does not actually touch the inner self. Just as a car driver involved in a minor fender-bender can get out and walk away without a scratch, the inner self can disconnect from the physical body and its various pains and sufferings.

The weakness of this automobile analogy is that a serious accident can hurt the driver. The inner self, however, is always aloof from the physical body in terms of the ability to survive and endure. While the self can be emotionally damaged (or educated) by the painful events of the physical world, the self will always come out without a scratch. The body may be burnt or thrown into a grave and buried after death, but the inner self can leave unscathed.

Detaching from Pain

The disconnection or detachment from pain on a temporary basis can be accomplished through the distraction of the self onto something other than the pain. This is certainly a bona fide strategy that is often utilized in hospitals. Emotional ties of this world, be it our family, a pet, the television, group events, or otherwise, can all provide temporary distraction and a subsequent reduction in the pain.

However, this will not provide an enduring solution, because these solutions are temporary. At some point, the family members and pets must leave, or die. The television must be turned off sooner or later. The group event must end and the group members must go home. All these solutions are fleeting. Once the distraction evaporates, we are left again to face our pain.

The long term solution is the detachment from the identification with this body and our expectations for future physical enjoyment. This means that we must give up the expectation that we will become fulfilled from the things of this world.

Those who hold on to this expectation of fulfillment from the physical world might say that this sure is a depressing outlook. This letting go of the expectation of fulfillment in the physical world will seem to them no different than giving up hope. They will say that what will get us through the pain will be the hope that the pain will go away and we will go on to live happy, fulfilling lives.

Certainly, projecting ahead to an expectation of no pain and physical fulfillment one day can distract us temporarily and even open up a greater possibility of physical healing. But this strategy can also result in depression, as we slowly realize that even if the pain lessens, we still have constant pain and it never seems to go away. In other words, the expectation that the pain will vanish and we will be eventually fulfilled through the physical body is a false hope: Every body is destined for pain and death.

What is better is a hopeful attitude that fulfillment can be found, and happiness can be found: just not in the physical world. If we see the physical world as a temporary place and we learn its lessons well, we can graduate to fulfillment. Then we not only have hope: We also have a realistic expectation of the future of the physical body and the potential of permanently leaving the pains of the physical world behind.

This does not mean that we will not still make an effort to heal the pain and get the body better. But the *reason* we do this will be different. We will be working to heal the body in order to use the body to further develop our spiritual evolution. And as we develop in our spiritual growth, we may become determined to use the physical body for a spiritual purpose (ergo, in the service of God). These activities give more than hope for fulfill-ment—they actually bring fulfillment.

This overall detachment is simply accomplished by realiza-tion. We can immediately become detached philosophically. We can realize that we are not these physical bodies. We can realize that our inner selves will live on, long after these physical bodies are rotting in their graves. We can realize that our happiness is based not on our physical condition, but upon our spiritual growth.

Once we achieve this simple philosophical realization, we can then move on towards practical realization. This means *act-ing* upon the knowledge that we are eternal and not these physi-cal bodies.

In other words, the greater our focus upon the higher pur-poses of life—such as spiritual growth and our relationship with God—the less sensitive we will be to the various aches and pains of the physical body. We will still feel these pains. We cannot simply wish them away. But because we will be refocused on a longer perspective, our current aches and pains will be under-stood as temporary. This might be compared again to the long distance runner who feels the pain, but knows that the pain is temporary. The runner knows as soon as the race is finished, the pain will be over. So they keep going, with their mind focused upon winning (or completing) the race.

Consider if we were on a boat and we were sailing towards a distant port. For many days, we will be focused on the condi-tions of the boat: what we are eating, the condition of the cabin, and so on. The boat is our main focus. Without the boat, the seas will swallow us. Then one day, we sight land. Suddenly, our perspective changes. We are no longer that interested in the daily minutia of the boat and its quarters. We are now glued to the binoculars as we determine where we are going to point the boat to arrive safely at port.

This is analogous to our situation as we approach the body's death. For decades, we have been focused upon every little whim of the body: When the body is hungry, we eat. When the body is tired, we sleep. When the body needs a bath, we take a bath. We follow the needs of the body around for many years, obeying its every beck and call. In other words, we have been focused on the body.

But now the body is aging and we are beginning to experience the aches and pains of the elderly years. We now are within sight of death. Or maybe we have been diagnosed with incurable cancer with less than a year to live. These are comparable to seeing a landfall: Death is within sight.

The pains of chronic disease indicate that we must now start broadening our horizon. We must look beyond the minutia of our physical bodies, and understand the greater meaning of life. We must carefully consider the death of the body, and begin to navigate our path beyond the body.

If we see each pain as lessons to be learned and as opportunities to evolve spiritually, we will gradually become detached to the body and learn to rise above pain. This does not mean we will not feel the pain. The pains will still be there. If we are fortunate, possibly the pain will even lessen a bit as we navigate our way towards port.

Pain is a purposeful signal that indicates a problem to fix and lessons to be learned. Certainly, our response to pain is best related to the type, location, and intensity of our pain. Some types of pain are more critical than others. These should be responded to with corrective measures if possible. For example, pain and numbness in the left arm or around the heart should be considered more critical than a sore thumb.

Pain medication may be necessary for some types of pain, but the goal of pain medication should be as a stopgap for a short period as a breather or to encourage the body to heal. Pain medication will likely not remove the cause of the pain. It can even increase the duration of the pain, as we can lose the incentive to remove the cause. If we can just take a pill and the pain goes away, we will neither learn from the pain nor learn how to remove the cause. Or if we know the cause, we may not develop the discipline needed to change our habits if it is easier just to take the pill. Pain medication may also cause dependency, and we will continuously need more to provide the same pain relief.

One of the best health professionals to approach for chronic pain is an acupuncturist. Clinical research on acupuncture has repeatedly shown it to be a successful treatment for pain of all types. Acupuncture has been used successfully for anesthesia for many centuries in China. Acupuncture has little risk and a long history of safety with little or no negative side effects. Acupuncture is a medical science and a medical art. The skill level of each practitioner and his or her connection with that type of pain might vary substantially. Therefore, we might consider going to another acupuncturist if one does not help before we give up altogether on acupuncture. Treatment cost is very low compared to other modalities, and success rates are high in many chronic pain disorders.

We should feel good about any treatment plan before we embark upon it. If we not feel comfortable with it, there is usually a good reason, and we might consider looking for an alternative. It is best to not ignore our intuition when it comes to healing. If we are not feeling comfortable, we should first probably discuss this with the health professional treating us at that time along with others. They may be able to remove our hesitations or provide an immediate alternative.

If we have some particular information gained from the internet or books about our treatment, we should present this to our health professional. We should at least fax or email the article or web pages and have the professional evaluate and respond to them. If they are not willing to do this, another professional should be approached to discuss these alternatives.

When seeing any professional for pain, we might also consider bringing in whatever supplements or medications we are taking, so they can look at the labels and consider what is already being taken before they prescribe others. This is a double concern for western medical doctors, as prescribing multiple medications with conflicting mechanisms has been occurring with greater frequency.

A pain diary is also very useful. We can rate our pain each day and see if the pain is increasing or decreasing, depending upon our diet, lifestyle and medication changes.

The bottom line is that we can empower ourselves during and between visits with health professionals. Empowerment strategies include keeping our own medical files, with a copy of every lab, x-ray and treatment plan in it. We can put into this file the medication information sheets (side effects) we are given; our pain and symptom diaries if we keep them; and any information or research data we gather relating to our pain or medical issue. We can bring this file into every health professional appointment to help substantiate our questions and concerns.

This file can prevent medical errors. When we bring our file to our visit, we can quickly access our information to show the health professional. This can greatly accelerate the quality of the information and advice we receive from our health professional.

At the end of the day, resolving our pain is our responsibility. Health professionals can offer advice and prescribe treatment, but we must be the ones who provide the effort and make the necessary changes.

Deathly Pain and Pain Medication

At some point in our lives, we will inevitably find our body in a situation of chronic disease and pain. Should we have the luxury of a clinical response, we will likely be presented with a treatment plan that includes aggressive painkillers. What do we do?

The decision to numb the body with painkillers should be made carefully. Painkillers should be used sparingly. They are a way to get through momentary periods of agony, but they can also lead us to vegetate into numbness if we are not careful. It is important to stay in touch with our body, because this is our contact with reality. Pain is our link to the awareness that we are not the body. Pain forces us to realize that the body is not an object of enjoyment. This is the quintessential 'teaching moment' of pain.

Without pain, we hide ourselves within a veil of illusion that the body is *me,* and the body will bring me pleasure. When we completely mask those moments when the body brings us pain with numbing medicines, we are not able to have this realization.

Most of us have heard our parents say as they disciplined us: *This is for your own good.* In other words, whatever the punishment, our parents *knew* that it was best for us. They knew somehow, that if we did not receive this punishment (hopefully not physical), we would not have the opportunity to learn something very valuable.

This is the same with occasional excruciating pain. Without feeling pain, we do not have the chance to understand the balance of our situation within the body. We do not get to understand that whether the body is feeling pleasure or feeling pain, we are the same. We are still the same person—able to observe that pain or pleasure.

People who have been through very painful periods in their lives can attest to this. They have come out of painful episodes with a deeper spiritual understanding of themselves. Quite often, as the pain began to get unbearable, they reached out for God.

Many have told us that after they reached out for God during these times, the found that God gave them relief. Even if the pain continued, they were able to bear it because God was there for them, comforting them internally. How else did they survive? This is evidenced by the many prisoner-of-war victims who have undergone torture and testified later that it was their faith in God that got them through the experience.

Should our prognosis be good and the cause of the pain is being resolved, temporary pain-relief may provide a bridge to the healing process. Should we be lost in numbness, however, the body's ability to resolve the issue will be decreased. Most health experts—even pain doctors—agree that pain drugs should be used as minimally as possible. This is a conclusion made from observation of thousands of patients who have succumbed to addictions and psychological defects as a result of aggressive painkillers.

Incredibly intense and chronic pain is likely a natural signal for the inner self to transition out of the physical body. With intense pain, the inner self is forced by necessity to disassociate with the body. This disassociation process is perfectly natural, and feeds the mechanism of the self separating from the body at death.

The message communicated with excruciating pain is that this temporary physical body is not our true identity—and the physical environment is not our true home. The reason we experience pain in the first place is because we are in conflict with our false ego. We are attempting to identify our self—the permanent emotional person—with a temporary vehicle. Acute chronic pain means the vehicle is becoming obsolete, through either injury or disease. And our desire for the survival of the body conflicts with this reality.

In other words, we have become attached to the body, and this attachment manifests itself as pain.

In order to 'evolve' beyond the body, we must become detached from it somehow. Pain naturally allows this to take place.

Some have proposed that pain is the imagination of the seer and therefore not real. Even those people who propose this will admit at some point that physical pain is very real. The body certainly undergoes damage, and during this damage, the nervous system communicates painful messages to the limbic system. These messages reflect onto the screen of the mind, allowing the inner self to experience it. The extent to which the inner self is attached to the body relates to the pain sensitivity as we've discussed. The messages from the body are real. The cause of the pain is real.

Consider for a moment watching a movie at a movie theater. As the movie plays on, you begin to associate and even identify yourself with the characters in the movie. Then suddenly, a tragedy befalls one of the characters. The character is in pain and suffering. Once you have associated with the character in the movie, you begin to 'feel his pain.' You become sensitive to the pains and suffering of the character. You might even wince as the hero gets attacked. Even though you know without a doubt that the character is simply an actor who is merely pretending to play the character and the actor is actually feeling no pain, you still become connected with the movie character's pain.

This is the same scenario experienced by the self. Even we realize theoretically that we are not the body, due to our lifelong association with the body, we will still be sensitive to the body's pain signals.

The difference is how we respond to the messages of pain. Both the attached person and the detached person will likely be sensitive to the body's pain. They will also both seek a solution to the pain. The difference lies to the *extent* each will go to obtain a solution to the pain.

The attached person will give anything for a solution. They will sacrifice anything—their integrity, purpose, or relationships with others. They will give up their deepest philosophical and religious feelings for the sake of relieving the pain.

A devoted person will respond differently. They will take action, but they will not sacrifice their core beliefs and mission to relieve the pain. This, in fact, is the traditional notion of martyrdom: If the devoted person is given the opportunity to die or give up their faith, they will choose death. This is vastly different, by the way, from the conception of some that martyrdom means to kill civilians along with committing suicide in the hopes of going to heaven. This is simply suicide and murder dressed up as religion.

The detached person will first focus on how to solve the problem caused by their pain. Failing that, they will transcend the pain with a focus on their true identity and purpose in this life. They will embrace the learning experience of the pain. They may stubbornly resist the pain. But they will never cross the line. They will embrace God's will. They will understand that whatever happens is part of God's plan.

Chapter Six

Our Time for Death

Each of our bodies will die at some point. No body makes it out alive. Most of us have two concerns about death: We wonder *when* we are going to die; and we wonder *what* will kill us.

Few of us consider what state will we be in when we die: What will we be focused on?

This is a critical question, because it is our consciousness at the time of death that determines our next destination.

The Biological Necessity of Death

The goal of modern medicine—and subsequently most health advice—is to help avoid the death of the body at all costs. Should this be our ultimate goal, however? The operator in this question is the *all costs* clause.

Families, patients and doctors typically struggle with the consequential questions: Just how much effort should be made to avert death? What is the point when death has its natural place, and we should accept its arrival? Should we continue to mount excessive costs and countless hours in a fruitless effort to try to prevent an eventuality? Does delaying death for a few days, weeks or months when there is little or no quality of life have any real value? Could it be a senseless and futile effort?

In June of 2006, the Centers for Disease Control released its annual report *Deaths: Preliminary Data for 2004*. This report showed a decrease in deaths in the United States by 3.9% from 2003. The 2003 report showed a decrease in deaths by 1.7% over 2002. This statistic is of course to be overlaid against the continued surging population of the United States during these years. In fact, this age-adjusted death statistic has been decreasing since 1900, with a few exceptions during disease outbreak years. This primarily means that over the past century, fewer babies die, and adults have been living longer in average years. In 2003, the average age of death was 77.5. Statistics show that 49 was the average lifespan in the United States at the turn of the twentieth century.

These can be a bit deceiving because a hundred years ago there were significantly more stillborns and more infant deaths. This skews the lifespan statistics. Many adults still lived to grand old ages, but the average between one stillborn and one *centenarian* (someone who lives to age 100) is close to 50 years old.

As far as diseases go, the number one cause of death in modern civilization has been heart disease, followed by cancer. Heart disease is a result of the modern diet. Over the past few years, cancer has overtaken heart disease as the leading killer. Higher cancer rates are of course connected to the chemical revolution of the past fifty years.

Due to the prevention education efforts and research focus of the American Heart Association and the American Cancer Society, death from these two diseases have been slightly decreasing over the past few years. Meanwhile, their occurrence appears to be increasing. While this could be attributed to greater diagnosis, it would ignore the fact that Americans are also becoming more obese; eating too much fried foods, junk food and meat. We might attribute the lower death rates to further advances in cardiovascular surgery (stents and so on) and chemotherapy—in addition to earlier diagnosis.

Our medical institutions are remarkable in their ability to artificially extend privileged patients' lives through intervention. In some cases, these heroic efforts may add a few quality years to a person's lifespan. In many cases, however, the intervention merely temporarily delays the inevitable. Those extended years are often spent drugged, numb, incapacitated and sometimes even unconscious.

Quite simply, death is a normal sequence of the self's occupancy within the body. It has the same importance to physical life that birth does. Death arrives at a time when the body is naturally becoming obsolete. As designed, the inner self exits when a significant portion of the body's major functions and organs break down. This is to our benefit. If we had to wait for all the parts of the body to break down before leaving, we would experience a greater amount of suffering. Instead, as soon as any of the major body parts—the brain, heart, liver, kidneys and so on—shuts down—the self is immediately escorted out of the body.

Every cell in the body has a programmed time to die. This genetic clock is subject to epigenetic change according to our activities, however. Cellular death is called *apoptosis*. Apoptosis can result from programmed death driven by internal clock or an external infliction that diseases the cell. Biologists have been investigating apoptosis' programmed processes over the past few decades, and have determined that cell death can occur through a combination of several signaling circuits.

One involves a programmed shutdown of the mitochondria (the energy production facilities of the cell), seemingly associated with the production of a signaling biochemical called the cytochrome-c. This signaling follows the development of a special signaling channel called the MAC (mitochondria apoptosis channel). The development of this special biocommunication channel appears mysterious. Still, we can surmise that this is simply part of the overall body's clockwork mechanism.

Scientists have also found that apoptosis often involves a complex process involving the internal self-destruct mechanism called tumor necrosis factor. The TNF mechanism was originally discovered in cancer research as the mechanism inhibiting the spread of a cancer. Researchers have since found that its process is related to several other mechanisms. These include the R1 and R2 receptor mechanisms. The R1 and R2 receptors receive signals from outside the cell to stimulate a process of shutting down the cell. The TNF signaling process instigates a cascading communication process called *death-induced signaling*. Here one signal to the R1 or R2 receptors stimulates a multi-instructional process that begins shutting down the cell. Part of this signaling process is transmitted through a genetic protein expression called the *p53 gene*. The p53 gene is a transcription protein affecting the process of genetic copying. Researchers have discovered that viruses and carcinogenic mutations are allowed to expand by disabling the p53 gene.

Another major signaling cell death mechanism is the *Fas-ligand* system. The Fas ligand is a specialized protein that signals to a receptor located on one of the chromosomes of the cell's DNA. This stimulation by the ligand—the signal-sending protein—seems to have its foundation in the T-cell immune system. As T-cells are activated, Fas ligands become more prolific, signaling the process of cell death.

In many circumstances, this also initiates the halting of mitosis—causing cells to die without replacements. In situations where a cell is infected by a virus or a carcinogenic mutation, the halting of mitosis can be inhibited by viral DNA mutations. By blocking the process of cell death, these viral mutations can multiply through cellular division. This of course allows the virus to replicate throughout the body—not a good scenario.

The apoptosis signaling process is still not well understood by medical science. The body's signalling mechanisms maintain that subtle programming feature scientists refer to as homeostasis. Homeostasis is sometimes used to describe cellular metabolism. Homeostasis also describes the body's ability to balance the number of cells that die with the number of new cells born through cellular division or mitosis. This balancing act is a complex programming feature. It cannot be unraveled by finding a few gene sequences. This process includes the expression of the p53 gene, the TNF process, various ligand-receptor mechanisms, and the overall mechanisms balancing the trillions of cells within the body. It becomes a macrocosm issue, and lies in the conscious epigenetic realm.

The ability of the body to orchestrate particular activities among the trillions of cells simultaneously to achieve governance over the body's major functions can only lie within the domain of greater design and consciousness—one requiring the master design of a superior intelligence.

The overriding message of these death-signaling mechanisms is that the body maintains a clock that times out the lifetimes of cells. As the body ages, dividing cells are outnumbered by dying cells. Living cells become less tolerant, and more prone to succumb to the challenges of our environment. At the same time, the immune system becomes more alert to challenged cells, responding quickly to eliminate cells that endanger the body during its remaining years.

These mechanisms all allow the self to proceed with its intentions of seeking fulfillment. We might compare this to the process of rationing. When a person knows that only so much food or water is left for a specific period of time, they will likely carefully divide up and measure each day's worth of the available food and water. In the same way, the design of the body continually accommodates the limitations of the body. As a result, the inner self seeks more conservative goals with modified expectations. Logically, the self could hardly expect fulfillment from reduced physical abilities. However, the false ego continues to tease the self with more concoctions of the mind in a futile expectation of physical fulfillment.

This seems curious, but we know it to be true. We see it in its most obvious form during a *mid-life crisis*. Here the self realizes that the body is quickly moving beyond a logical hope that certain physical functions will continue. This presents a conflict of identity: The body is getting old but the inner self feels the same age. In a desperate attempt to reconcile this conflict, the misidentifying self may instigate a radical move. We have seen many examples of this. A person might purchase a motorcycle, re-enter a former sport, try to have a baby, or attempt to date someone younger.

The inner self adapts to age by accommodating these physical changes with redirected expectations. Instead of expecting fulfillment by winning a football game, the aging star will seek fulfillment by coaching a victorious team. In both efforts, the goal has not changed. In both, the self is seeking the approval and love from others.

As the body ages further, the self begins to lose the opportunities to accomplish anything significantly physical. The inner self may then redirect expectations for physical fulfillment in the accomplishments of the body's children or grandchildren. When the child or grandchild succeeds, they feel that they succeed.

Just as did the physical accomplishments, this also does not fulfill the inner self. We know this scientifically because we can observe successful parents and grandparents still plagued by loneliness, panic-attacks and a general lack of fulfillment—despite the collective achievements of their children and grandchildren.

A Timely Message

The dying of the body has a clear message: It is time for us to exit. We have arrived at a point where the lessons of this lifetime should have been learned. Now it is time for a new journey. It is time for us to move on.

Death is like being shown the door. When we are visiting with friends at their house and our hosts suddenly get up from the sofa and begin to slowly walk towards the door, we know it is time to leave. It is time to thank our host for their hospitality, and move on. It is not time to start up another conversation. Or go back and sit on the sofa. Should we do this, we will probably be accused of overstaying our welcome.

This is not too dissimilar to the scenario playing out in most hospitals today.

The natural body is simply not designed to live forever. This is observable by any scientific study. Yet our modern medical institutions tease us with notions of new technologies that might keep the body alive forever.

We should know this will happen. Nor is it a good use of our precious time while still here. The laws of nature have a reason. We inhabit a physical body for a short time to learn specific lessons. It is a short-term vehicle. The body is not meant to house the living being forever. It is like putting on a spacesuit with a particular oxygen reserve. Once within the temporary spacesuit, a smart astronaut does not waste time debating about why there is not more oxygen in the tank. It is what it is, and the astronaut has a particular job to do before returning to the space ship.

The problem is that we falsely identify with the physical body after a few years in it. This is also by design. Once this mis-identification grabs us—which happens pretty early on in our lives in this body—we become connected to the body. We try to protect it at all costs. We scream when it becomes threatened. We raise our hackles when a life-threatening challenge presents itself.

We have discussed how the inner self can be deceived by the body's stress chemicals. Our body can be pumping out emergency biochemicals and signals even when little is at stake. This misinterpretation can also be evident during a truly life-threatening situation. We have often seen situations where people become so anxious during a traumatic experience that they do not react appropriately. We might do the wrong thing under the circumstances. We might scream when in reality no one can hear us or help us. We might freeze like a deer in the headlights when we should be running from a threat.

During the 9/11 disaster, some people reacted calmly and intelligently during the disaster. They evacuated in an orderly fashion while helping others. Meanwhile, more people panicked and did not act appropriately. Most of us agree that an over-stimulated panic state can sometimes be a distraction or even a deterrent from dealing with an emergency. For this reason, most of us consider a state of panic with disdain. We also admire those who coolly and calmly react during a crisis.

Why do we respect those who calmly react appropriately in a crisis? This is because most of us see a panic response as being disconnected from the reality of an emergency. An overstated panic response is often seen in groups. A panicked group of people can easily over-react and over-step the boundaries of what should be done. This is often because these people are watching everyone else's response rather than assessing the situation directly.

As a result, they are out of touch with the problem and tend to react as others do. Research has shown that in an emergency, crowds tend to spontaneously select a group leader or role model—often arbitrarily. As the inherited leaders of the group respond, the rest of the group is likely to respond similarly. Should these 'chosen ones' react inappropriately, the entire crowd follows suit. Suddenly the situation becomes a crisis because an entire group or population of people is responding inappropriately to a perceived threat. We might call this the *herd mentality*.

This is precisely the situation existing today amongst our medical institutions with regard to the process of death.

It is appropriate to respond urgently to a patient who has been shot or critically injured. Attempts are made to extract the bullet or repair the injury. These are acceptable responses to a critical injury that may easily be healed with intervention. Heroic attempts to resuscitate a younger individual who has had a heart attack or stroke might be considered appropriate as well.

There is a critical line, however, between these types of emergency interventions and unacceptable attempts to intervene in the natural process of death. The line becomes evident when the body is chronically malfunctioning, and chronic pain without medication has become unbearable.

As we have discussed previously, tens of thousands of near-death experiences have documented accurate recollections after the clinical death of the body. Most documented clinical death experiences include the self first floating up over the body and looking down upon it. At this point, the self can observe the physical events taking place around the body. The self may observe the doctors and nurses operating or attempting resuscitation. Many have traveled into the hallways and into other rooms to observe other events. Thousands of these unembodied observations have been recalled following resuscitation. Furthermore, practically every viewing experience that could be checked was confirmed as accurate. In other words, there are no known cases where the observations of the unembodied self have proven to be inaccurate.

Think about it. This is physically impossible for a body lying in a bed unconscious, with their eyes closed, and brain dead. Many cases document the unembodied self instantly traveling to remote locations to see friends or relatives. They might look upon a relative or spouse in an attempt to say goodbye. Once again, most of these accurately describe the activities and even clothing of this distant relative. How could the self have accurately observed the activities of their relative if their body was lying clinically dead in a hospital bed thousands of miles away?

Most NDE experiences report entering a tunnel with a light at the other end. Many have reported meeting with a spiritual personality. Many have also reported being informed by this individual that it was "not their time yet." This was typically followed by the immediate return of the self to the body.

A significant number of clinical death patients have had these experiences. Dr. Kubner-Ross and her associates, whose research we mentioned earlier, studied approximately 20,000 cases of clinical death.

Note these studies of clinical death or near death experiences have been conducted with scientific scrutiny and peer review. Many were controlled to specifically address concerns made from previous clinical death studies. Some of the researchers—many of whom were medical doctors—were doubtful about life after death prior to their research. By the end of their research, most became convinced of life after death.

While there is still some debate surrounding the meaning of these studies, the evidence is clear. During clinical death, not only has the heart stopped and breathing stopped: Brainwaves have also stopped. This means there is little or no electrical activity in the body. If consciousness were part of the electrical activity of the brain as some contend, then the observations of the patient would have also stopped at the same time. Instead, those experiences continued for a significant percentage of clinically dead patients.

It should be pointed out that there were also many clinical death subjects who do not recall the death experience. Suicide and drug-overdose subjects, for example, typically have no recollection. For others, the excess of painkillers, psychotic medications or simply an incoherent state of mind likely block the recollection of the experience upon awakening.

This might be compared to our ability to recall dreams. Most of us do not recall our dreams. Occasionally we do. When we do, we consider it an extraordinary situation. In the same way, the near-death experience is a completely different state of awareness. Not remembering this state with the conscious mind should not be considered so unusual.

The self has innate consciousness and memory, but this level of awareness is easily blocked by the mind's restrictions. This is illustrated by Dr. Stevenson's research with regression among children. Many young children can remember their past lives, but this recollection typically fades after the age of seven—as the mind's architecture begins to block out those memories.

For those thousands that remember their NDEs, the state of awareness was altogether different than dreaming or physical life. This does not mean they were not aware of the circumstances of their body's death. Many observed and accurately recalled actual events as they occurred around their deathbed or accident location—during a time when their bodies were clinically dead. Some cases have documented that the clinically-dead person was able to rise above the fray and see (and recall) the accurate license plate of the hit-and-run car that nearly killed their body.

Despite the clarity of these studies, some steadfast doubters have proposed that the clinical death experience is nothing but mental hallucination. This might be plausible if not for the fact that hallucinations are defined as seeing something that *did not happen*. Since a number of researchers have confirmed that the observations made by the clinically dead were accurate, the hallucination theory would not be plausible. Indeed, many have based their arguments on an assumption that consciousness originates in the brain. If the brain was electrically dead—as it was in many of these clinical death cases—then how could the person be conscious during that time?

Dr. Kübler-Ross' research meticulously eliminated all the factors that her peers presented as possible explanations (outside of the self leaving the body). Some have suggested that the experiences were mental projections of what might happen. For these, Dr. Kübler-Ross studied cases of blind people who were blind from birth, and/or had no light reception for at least the past ten years. Many of these viewed accurate colors among clothing, walls and other objects during their observations after being clinically dead. They, like the others, also recalled seeing family members in remote locations while their body was lying clinically dead in the hospital bed. Furthermore, the recollections of the resuscitated person were made even though the resuscitated physical body of the person was still blind.

The only logical explanation to be gained from this research is that we are not the physical body. Rather, each of us has an identity transcendental to the body. The physical body we wear is merely a temporary vehicle. This is a truly scientific position, noting also that the body undergoes so many physical changes over a lifetime while we remain *ourselves*. The body is recycling cells and molecules while the personality within remains the same personality.

With these realities in mind, we can be certain that death is simply our leaving a worn-out vehicle and moving on. Where we go is the appropriate discussion.

So we must now ask this important question: Knowing the body will inevitably become obsolete and will eventually die, and we will live beyond this death, why should we respond inappropriately to the prospect of death? Why should we unnaturally keep a person from the next step in their journey, and keep them in a state of suspension? Certainly, there is little quality of life in living out a few months in a hospital bed attached to life-support equipment and unable to conduct meaningful physical or mental activities.

Certainly, doctors are not feeling improper while they valiantly rescue a dying person. In many cases, they are not being improper either. However, we all know examples of situations where their efforts become ridiculous. Most of us have heard of cases where a person is kept on resuscitating equipment well past a reasonable period of time. The patient remains unconscious, and without the equipment the body would surely cease existing. At this point, the inner self is trapped and not being let go. The self is stuck without the ability to communicate or request to be let go. This is simply unfair and cruel.

Note that we are not making a determination here of where the line should be drawn, or isolating which types of resuscitation are reasonable. This is a personal decision that should be made by each of us. Each of us is responsible for the efforts that others make on behalf of our body. Therefore each of us is responsible for making the determination for the limitation of heroic efforts, and making this clear (in writing) to our relatives and health professionals. In the absence of this, it will become the decision of our spouse or relatives.

This is a very difficult position to be in as a relative. Any caring spouse or family member will struggle with such a decision, because they do not want their mate or relative to leave them. They also will be presented with the appearance, possibly, of wanting to hasten the death of their spouse. Putting our spouse or relatives in this position is simply unfair. Sometimes, in the absence of clear instructions by the dying person, a court or legislative body will become involved in the decision of whether to disconnect the person from their life-support equipment.

Why should we put others in such an uncomfortable position? Why should we involve total strangers in the decision about whether we wish to be let go or not?

This is not to say that while we occupy the physical body we should not be working to keep our body in good condition as long as it is useful. Keeping the body in good condition will allow it to run efficiently and effectively. Certainly if we do not treat the body well, we will be condemned to dealing with the consequences of ill health. Ill health in this situation is also part of nature's design for learning.

Once our bodies have played out their intended era, it is not the time to focus on attempts to avoid death at all costs. It is a time to embrace death as a natural progression of our physical journey. It is time for us to consider the meaning of life and death. It is a time to begin transcending the physical layers of the body and mind. It is time to achieve a higher understanding about our existence.

This is the purpose of old age. During our elderly years, we can no longer look towards any career advancement. We cannot achieve sexual prowess. We are done planning for our future retirement. We have little ability to train for winning a sporting event. We can certainly keep active through our elderly years. However, we must accept our elderly years as a period of weakened physical abilities. These are the years to focus on and prepare for our transition out of the body.

Instead, our health care industry and society works with great difficulty to distract the elderly from this mission. For this reason, pharmaceutical drug use is rampant among the elderly. The elderly are often distracted in nursing homes with meaningless games, television and mind-altering drugs. Activity and social events may certainly have some positive attributes, and some drugs may be required for certain circumstances. But the importance of a clear mind to use for spiritual contemplation and reflection should be tantamount during these years.

Our medical institution's attempts to extend life are useless. Certainly, we have been able to extend the lifetime of people's bodies in some respects with our medical technologies. We have been able to transplant hearts, install stents and replace kidneys. What are the costs of these efforts? Are all these technologies really extending the quality of our lives? Is there a net gain after we consider the time spent on the effort? Some transplants might be reasonable. Others can be risky and ultimately doomed for failure.

Let's compare this effort to the logic we might use when deciding whether to drive or fly to a destination. We would compare the driving and stopping time to the airport waits, the flight, and the travel to and from the airport. Sometimes a drive might be faster than a flight, or the flight might be faster and even cheaper than the drive after gas and meals are considered.

The quality of our remaining life can be analyzed similarly. In measuring the cost of prolonging life, we have to net out how much time is taken by doctor's visits, hospitalization, surgery, recuperation, rehabilitation, and the various follow-up visits. Then we must consider the risks and side effects involved in the treatment. This risk and treatment time needs to be subtracted from the extra days or years gained from the treatment. We should also subtract the time spent deciding on the treatment, researching the treatment and so on. All of this time spent looking to avoid death should be subtracted from the net conscious time gained in order to assess the value of the treatment. This relates directly to the quality of life achieved. If the process leaves us unable to return to our families and lifestyle in a reasonable amount of time then what good was all the effort?

Included in this consideration is how much of the doctors' time is being taken away from the efforts of saving those who can have a longer lifespan. Consider the children who are dying of malaria, AIDS and other ailments. With the kind of cost and focus put upon the medicine for extending the lives of the end-of-life stage elderly, more of these children could be treated.

We should also consider in this evaluation the many billions of dollars and time resources spent by many researchers, doctors, professionals, hospitals, pharmaceutical companies and insurance providers; all aimed at attempting to add a few days, months or a year or two to lives that have already lasted 70 or 80 years. Is it worth all this human effort?

The United States' economy is drowning in medical costs. The current head of the Government Accounting Office admits that the cost of health care and pharmaceuticals in the United States will bankrupt Medicare and possibly the entire government within a decade or two. Health care costs have risen from 4% of America's gross national product in 1950 to a whopping 16% in 2004. And 25% of Medicare costs in the U.S. are spent during the last year of life, and 10-12% are spent during the last two weeks of life.

Currently the U.S. is number one in the world for per-capita spending on healthcare, yet ranked number fifty-eight for longevity. Obviously much of our spending and resources is going to waste. What if we were to put all of the money, energy and resources we spend trying to unnaturally stay alive towards caring for and preventing childhood sickness, and feeding hungry people around the world? We would probably live in a much kinder world, and become better prepared to leave it. We would probably also all live longer, as we would likely have less stress—a central cause of a majority of fatal diseases. The bottom line with this point is that a consciousness of kindness also makes our bodies healthier.

What Happens when My Body Dies?

The research of Dr. Moody, Dr. Kübler-Ross, Dr. Sabom, Dr. Ring and others has given us a clear scientific understanding of what happens when we die. Thousands of clinical death patients have come back to tell us what is on the other side. Their information is invaluable. With it, we can combine some of the peer-reviewed hypnosis research and the ancient knowledge applicable to this. Together this allows us to present, from a scientific basis, what will happen to each of us when we die:

First, some event will shock our body into the sequence of dying. This may be a heart attack, a stroke or a fatal accident. At the point of death, our heart will malfunction and our brain will be deprived of oxygen and glucose. This will induce brain death. We will feel numbness throughout the body. As this happens, our bodies will become unconscious, and we will slip out of the body via one of the body's orifices.

We will rise above our body. As we rise, we will have a sense of exhilaration as we realize that we are still alive. We will be overjoyed knowing that we are fully intact, and whatever physical handicaps we had within the body will no longer constrain us. For example, if our bodies were in a wheelchair, we will be amazed that we can suddenly dance and walk. If our bodies were blind, we will be overjoyed to find that we can see in full color and definition.

During this phase, we have left our gross physical body but have retained our ethereal body. The ethereal body retains our projection of false ego that defined the shape of our gross physical body. Therefore, we still identify with the gross physical body and feel that we are still within our own dimension.

We are floating above our body, watching the events occurring around it. We watch as urgent care specialists try to revive the body. We watch as our family members gather around to mourn our loss. We begin to speak to them. We tell them that we are okay. We tell them that we are still alive.

After a few minutes of communicating to them we realize that they do not hear us. They do not know we are standing right next to them or above them, trying to speak to them. While we are elated to be alive, this is a little disappointing.

If our relatives or loved ones are not around our body at the time of death, we will go to them. At the speed of thought we will immediately be at their side where ever they are. They might be halfway around the world. We will still be there in an instant. Again we will be next to them or floating above, watching them. They might be crying or otherwise engaged in mourning our departure. We are a bit frustrated with this, as we try to communicate to them that we are still here.

Soon we realize that although we are alive, our body and this environment is no longer our home. We are moving on.

We are now signaled by our guardian angel that it is time to move on. We are drawn into a passageway that may be described as tunnel (some describe it as a river or mountain pass). Suddenly we are being pulled through this passageway. The tunnel represents our transitional exit from the physical dimension and our ethereal body. At the end of the tunnel is a dazzling light. As we arrive into this lit area, we find ourselves in the presence of one or several of God's representatives (angels). They are beautiful, kind and also dazzle with light and spiritual energy. If we have developed a relationship with God during our lifetime, God Himself may be present.

At this location we suddenly have full awareness. We no longer have a body or mind. We are pure spirit, yet we still have all our faculties of feelings and emotions. We are awestruck and humbled by the experience.

Our entire physical life is flashed back in front of us in an instant. We understand that the body was an educational vehicle, and we were supposed to have learned certain lessons. We see in an instant every decision we made during that physical lifetime. We see every event and every purposeful impact we had upon others. We see the love we shared, and the love we took. We see the anger, the violence, and the poor judgment. At the same time, we see the good decisions we made that helped others. We are peering at our lives as though it was a microscope allowing us to instantly see everything we did along with their consequences. We are saddened by actions that hurt others, and gladdened by actions that helped others.

While this flashback was intended for our review, it is also accompanied by a judgment from God (if present) or God's representative(s). While we understand that the judgment has already been made, it is displayed before us in order for us to understand its perfection. The judgment takes into account all of our decisions, consciousness and desires as a whole, and sums them into a direction and location to move on to.

We instantly understand that the judgment given is a fair one. For as our physical life is flashed back, we can see our delinquencies and deficiencies. In the presence of God's representative we can clearly understand the areas that need improvement. This understanding naturally evolves into the decision of where we go next.

While this decision is not ours, we do indeed participate. This is accomplished because of the love and compassion of God's representatives. As they communicate the judgment, we see its wisdom.

Where we go depends upon the activities of our physical lives. It depends upon the condition of our consciousness. As we lived within the body, we developed certain tendencies. These might be violence, animosity, jealousy and anger. Or they might be wisdom, compassion and curiosity. In the former case, we are directed to giving birth in a new physical body. This might be the physical body of a violent animal: One that can express our anger with fewer restrictions.

Or in the later case, we might move on to another human form: one that will allow us to further develop our spiritual growth while at the same time reaping the results of our activities — good and bad. Regardless, we realize it is a perfect system, and accept our fate.

For the person being reborn into an animal or lower body, there might be a great reluctance. The representatives of God who display our judgment may suddenly become its enforcers.

We may struggle with our destination but they bind us and deliver us to the lower kingdom, as sperm traveling to the egg of a beast. Here we begin a downward spiral, from one beastly body to the next, suffering the karma of our human activities. We descend from beast to beast in successive lives, dropping even to insect and bacteria levels, before finally—possibly after millions of lifetimes in various lower species—again having the opportunity of a human lifetime.

For extreme cases, it is possible that we are not even delivered to the transition platform for our judgment. Our judgment may be immediately given as we enter the tunnel; where our lives are flashed before us as we move to the tunnel's exit and directly into the sperm of our next species.

Alternatively, we may arrive at 'judgment day' in a spiritually advanced state. This is the person who spent a significant part of their lives (or even the last part) perfecting their relationship with God. They utilized the teachings of the masters and scripture to advance to a point where they had re-developed their loving relationship with the Supreme Person and His children.

This sort of person dies quite differently. In this case, we are immediately greeted by God's representatives upon death. These happy angels embrace and begin to escort us. They arrive with a beautiful chariot. We humbly step into the chariot, and it is whisked away, through the tunnel and through the depth of the space of dazzling light. As we enter this region, we are greeted by countless angels—most of whom we know intimately for some reason. We are embraced and welcomed by all. As we arrive at our spiritual destination, we are brought before our beautiful and ever-youthful God, where we have the opportunity to humbly honor Him. As we are honoring Him, He picks us up and embraces us. *"Welcome home,"* He says lovingly, full of compassion and forgiveness for our humble feelings of failure and inadequacy.

Dying in the Hospital

Most people do not want to die in the hos
time, most people do not want to die period. S
ing to the hospital in the hopes of being save
dying there.

So we now have another calculation to make: Do we risk going to the hospital? Is it worth the risk? This decision is one that
should be made between the individual, their physician and
their spiritual advisor. The analysis should include the facts, as
well as a judgment call on whether our illness is treatable in the
long run.

'Treatable in the long run' simply means that the fix from the
hospital renders a significant amount of independent mobility
for a significant amount of time. A treatment that requires a person to stay on a heart and lung machine for the rest of his or her
life should not be considered much independent mobility, for
example. Or a transplant that gives the patient one extra week of
life should not be considered a significant amount of time.

In between these lies a large grey area, however. One that
only the patient should decide upon, taking into account the risk
of the treatment. If we are going to undergo a transplant to add
one week to our body's life, and the surgery runs a great risk of
failure, perhaps this is not such a great strategy.

Again this is highly personal, because we might have a project we badly need to complete before we die and if we don't get
the surgery we will surely die within a day or two. Or perhaps
the heart and lung machine will allow us a little time to complete
a particular task.

Often it is a risk/analysis equation. One example is the
breast mammogram. A 2008 study out of Holland confirms that
they exert about 1,000 times the radiation exposure as a chest x-
ray and directly increase the risk of breast cancer. Yet research
shows they provide little benefit in the way of early cancer detection compared to the manual breast examinations by physicians.

Much of the advances in technology have come in the way of various life-extension systems such as feeding tubes, ventilators, dialysis machines and heart-lung equipment. Today ones body can easily become a surrogate of one of these machines long after the intended time of death has past. Furthermore, the cost of putting someone on these extravagant machines bankrupts thousands of American families every year.

Interestingly, many of these new technologies and medicines create as many early deaths as they may temporarily prevent. The statistics show that our medical institution has become the leading cause of death and injury in the United States. Carolyn Dean, M.D., N.D., in her book, *Death By Medicine* (2005), compiled the following statistics for 2005:

Adverse Reactions	106,000 Deaths
Medical Errors	98,000 Deaths
Bedsores	115,000 Deaths
Hospital Infections	88,000 Deaths
Outpatient Adverse Reactions	199,000 Deaths
Unnecessary Procedures	37,136 Deaths
Surgery-Related	32,000 Deaths
Total Deaths	**783,936 Deaths**

Think about this. This accounting of deaths out-numbers U.S. cardiovascular disease deaths and cancer deaths. In 2002 for example, 450,637 people died of heart disease and about 476,009 died of cancer.

The *Journal of the American Medical Association* (Lazarou *et al.* 1998) reported that in 1994, 2,216,000 Americans were either hospitalized, permanently disabled, or died as a result of pharmaceuticals. *The Nutrition Institute of America* reports that over 20 million unnecessary antibiotic prescriptions are prescribed. Over seven million medical and surgical procedures a year are unnecessary. Over eight million people are hospitalized without need. Our medical institution is quite simply suffocating in its own mismanagement.

Note that Lazarou's research indicated that over 2.2 million Americans annually with *reported* injuries from pharmaceuticals.

The study, done at the University of Toronto, also showed that approximately 106,000 people die each year from taking *correctly prescribed* FDA-approved pharmaceuticals. This does not include the number of deaths resulting from the illegal sale and overdose of these same drugs.

The U.S. FDA was sent 258,000 adverse drug events in 1999. Harvard researcher and associate professor of medicine Dr. David Bates told the *Los Angeles Times* in 2001 *"...these numbers translate to 36 million adverse drug events per year"* (Rappoport 2006). The plausibility of this number is confirmed in another study published in the *Journal of the American Medical Association* in 1995 (Bates *et al.*). This revealed that over a sixth month period, 12% of 4031 adult hospital admissions had either a confirmed adverse drug event or a potentially adverse drug event. If we extrapolate this rate using the population of 300 million Americans, we would arrive at the 36 million Rappoport calculated.

According to a nationwide poll conducted by Louis Harris and Associates released in 1997 by the National Patient Safety Foundation and the American Medical Association, an estimated 100 million Americans experienced a medical mistake: 42% of those randomly surveyed. Misdiagnosis and wrong treatments accounted for 40% of those mistakes. Medical medication errors accounted for 28% of these, and medical procedure errors accounted for 22% of these 100 million medical mistakes (NPSF 1997).

In a study of four Boston adult primary care practices involving 1202 outpatients, 27% (95% confidence) of responders experienced adverse drug events (Gandhi *et al.* 2003).

In a 2004 interview with Dr. Lucian Leape, an expert in patient safety and an author of a number of studies, reported that over the past ten years since the 1997 NPSF studies were performed, improvements in our medical system have been inadequate. Barriers to improvement cited physician denial, hospital environment, lack of leadership and little system review (Leape 2004).

As we settle back into our seats after reading these startling facts, we should realize that this means our medical institutions' supposed heroic endeavors for life extension actually cost more lives than they save. These efforts actually shorten more lives than they extend. To add insult to injury, the dramatically rising cost of medical care in our society also means less access to medical care for preventive care and non-critical treatment. In real terms, this means that poorer people and the uninsured receive less healthcare, while preventive healthcare receives little or no attention.

Our medical institutions' supposed heroic effort to save lives is backfiring. Why? Because pharmaceutical and medical technology companies are madly pursuing profits while medical doctors are over-prescribing pharmaceuticals and over-applying diagnostic procedures in an attempt to avoid malpractice suits. The situation is not dissimilar to a large herd of confused animals stampeding and mowing down anything in the way.

For those who believe America's advanced healthcare technologies are extending lives, we only have to point to the statistics. The United States has one of the lowest life expectancies among the industrialized world, while leading the world in the application of the newest technologies and healthcare costs. Meanwhile we see people living very longer in places like Okinawa and Tibet, where medical technology and advanced drugs are less available.

We have traded in our blue skies for asbestos ceiling tiles and our sun for fluorescent lights. We traded air for soot and food for sugar and preservatives. The increases in life expectancy in the industrialized countries are due primarily to increased live birth rates and dramatic end-of-life procedures that add little in the way of quality of life.

As a result, there has been a major shift in the types of diseases modern man is faced with. Third world countries and traditional cultures are faced with death from infectious epidemics and birth deaths. Western society, however, is challenged by a myriad of autoimmune disorders, cancers, heart disease and nervous disorders.

Modern medicine has valiantly challenged many infectious diseases with vaccination and antibiotics. The jury is still out, however, on whether these strategies will ultimately free us from infectious disease. With the rampant growth of antibiotic-resistant superbugs like methicillin resistant *Staphylococcus aureus* (MRSA) and antibiotic-resistant tuberculosis, our fight against infectious disease is far from over. As infectious organisms learn how to counteract our antibiotics, the number of superbugs are growing. This all but eliminates any expectation of dominance over infectious disease.

As a result of modern medicine's advancements, our doctors feel like superheroes when they extend the life of a person's body temporarily. This is regardless of the quality of life remaining with the patient. The quality of life for an elderly person undergoing multiple operations, medications, life-support equipment and repeated hospitalization is significantly limited. Is it worth it?

These heroic efforts to 'save lives' by doctors are certainly valiant. Many activities in private medicine are motivated simply by profits, however. Pharmaceutical companies and healthcare organizations are generally multi-billion dollar enterprises built upon a mission of profitability. Their stockholders, directors, and management are thus focused upon making profitable decisions. This creates an obvious conflict of interest.

Once a pharmaceutical company has designed new drug, it can receive patent protection for that chemical combination, giving the company twenty years of potential exclusivity for selling that drug, at least in the United States.

However, without a doctor to prescribe the medication, there is no continual use of the drug. For this reason, pharmaceutical companies employ extensive marketing teams and budgets. They have also been known to fund lavish conferences at tropical resorts for prescribing doctors, along with free meals and other perks.

Pathology courses in western medical schools also accompany instruction on prescribing specific pharmaceutical drugs. The institution synchronizes with the pharmaceutical industry because of the tight relationships between pharmaceutical companies, medical schools, medical licensure and pathology course materials. Drug research is often conducted at medical schools, which retain funding from pharmaceutical manufacturers. There is thus a built-in incentive for medical schools to teach pharmaceutical-oriented medicine.

A number of recent reports and lawsuits have indicated that pharmaceutical-sponsored studies have not disclosed critical side effects some drugs. We have also seen that some doctors have been exposed for signing off on fraudulent or incomplete research data. Multiple reports have indicated that doctors paid to sign off on research never even looked at the raw data. Pharmaceutical-sponsored research is now turned down by the *Journal of the American Medical Association* for these reasons, yet many other journals accept pharmaceutical-company sponsored research. One study concluded that pharmaceutical company-paid researchers were significantly less likely to report adverse side effects from the drugs made by their employers.

Even if a pharmaceutical drug results in an improved condition for a particular ailment, there can often be dangerous side effects. Some of these can be worse than the original ailment. In addition, most medications stress the liver and kidneys in one respect or another — shortening the lifespan of these critical organs. Some medications, including aminoglycoside antibiotics streptomycin, kanamycin, garamicin and others have been shown to cause kidney damage in as many as 15 percent of patients. Others, such as acetaminophen, carbamazepine, atenolol, cimetidine, phenylbutazone, acebutolol, piroxicam, mianserin, naproxen, sulindac, ranitidine, enflurane, halothane, valproic acid, phenobarbital, isoniazid and ketoconazole can cause acute dose-dependent liver damage.

This is because the liver and the kidneys work together to process most chemicals out of the body. Together these organs break down and excrete the chemical byproducts of medications, resulting in their hopeful extraction from the body. With this chemical breakdown comes a number of dangerous residual chemical derivatives. For example, the P450 liver enzyme process moves chemicals through the extraction pathway. This enzyme is effective in most healthy bodies for a few chemicals at a time. Multiple drugs can overwhelm and deplete this pathway. With the P450 extraction pathway overloaded by various chemicals, additional drugs can more significantly damage the body. For this reason, a higher number of liver enzymes in a blood analysis is seen by doctors as a dangerous sign.

Sadly, multiple drug prescribing is commonplace among the elderly. In America, a large number of elderly persons (especially those who regularly see a doctor) are taking multiple medications. A 2004 Duke University study showed that 21% or 7 million Americans over the age of 65 take drugs classified as "dangerous." The over-65 population is 15% of the overall population, and this group is taking one-third of all drug prescriptions. Study researchers added that the study actually understated the problem, and that an elderly person taking at least ten to twelve prescription drugs at a time is common.

What this translates to is an elderly population being drugged through their "golden years." Because doctors are prescribing multiple mood-altering drugs to this group of people, we are left with a growing population of elderly drug-dependency. Suddenly drugs have become necessary for sleep. Drugs have become needed to eat. Drugs have become needed to maintain composure. Drugs have become needed to get through the day.

Why has our elderly become increasingly drug-dependent? Primarily because elderly people become vulnerable as they begin to face their many physical failings and impending death. After a lifetime of physical activity and an assumption that life was going to last forever, the elderly have become insecure about identity and old age. This is a byproduct of educational institutions that ignore the science of our true identity.

Impressed by the physician's credentials and the prolific advertising of the pharmaceutical industry, it is quite easy to be convinced of the necessity of taking these drugs. Drug advertising aimed at the elderly will typically show elderly people laughing, enjoying life and being active. This creates the message that the drug will help make us happy. Advertisers increasingly imply that drugs will create fulfillment and quality of life during a time meant for contemplation and introspection.

We must turn this equation around. At a time when a person needs to have clarity and purpose of mind, our medical institutions are drugging us and tempting us with unrealistic expectations. As we approach the crossroads of our physical journey — and begin our transition from this body to our next destination — we need to be prepared for the true healing event.

What is the reason for dying? Dying is the process of learning the 'take-away points' from a lifetime of lessons stemming from our life's challenges, pain, laughter, love, relationships, losses and gains. More importantly, it is the knowledge and wisdom we've gained as we leave it all behind.

At this time more than any, we need to utilize all our faculties in order to navigate this important step in our existence.

In other words, we must preserve our awareness as we take this important next step. Let's compare this to stepping into a new building for the first time. We have never been in this building, so we are not sure where the steps are, where the elevator is, or where a particular hallway will lead us. So when we enter the building, we need to be keenly aware of our surroundings. We need to be focused on where we will be going, or we may end up at the end of a long hallway without an exit.

In the same way, as we prepare to step through the doorway of death, we need to have our wits about us. We need to be as aware and prepared as possible. There are several strategies we can use to help accomplish this.

Managing our Body's Death

One consideration is putting in place a *living will*. The living will can detail our wishes for how our body is maintained if we are no longer able to communicate those decisions directly. The living will can therefore contain detailed instructions on health treatments we would consider acceptable with regard to critical care and ambulatory resuscitation.

For example, the living will may instruct whether life support equipment is to be connected in the event we become unconscious. It may also detail specific instructions, such as whether feeding tubes, heart-lung machines, ventilators or other equipment is to be employed. We can detail whether blood transfusions, transplants and other care is acceptable to us, and if so, to what extent or for how long. It can also be specific as to what types of medications are acceptable to us, and if so, how long those medications should be sustained. The living will should specify our wishes on critical care treatment with the greatest of clarity and detail.

A critical part of the living will is the appointment of a *health care advocate.* The health care advocate is a person we trust to oversee our health care treatment should we become hospitalized or incapacitated. This person is also given the ability to make certain decisions on our behalf. Therefore, this person needs to be someone we trust implicitly to carry out our instructions as they are recorded in our living will.

Specific instructions regarding emergency medical treatment are often called *advance medical directives.* In such a situation where we are deemed unable to make our own decisions, these instructions must be followed. It is therefore important that our health care advocate have a copy of this living will so that he or she can show it to doctors and hospital administrators in the case of a our need for emergency treatment. This means alerting the person that they are our advocate, and keeping our living will in a reasonably accessible location. In the U.S. attorneys are often the caretakers of these documents. They are required by their bar license to keep them on file and as safe as possible, and disclose them to whom the directives indicate upon request or circumstance. *(The comments here are not legal advice. Consult a legal professional for specific advice regarding the living will, advanced medical directives, health advocate and/or other solutions.)*

Without advance medical directives or such a living will, we could be given medications we cannot or do not want to physically, mentally, emotionally or spiritually tolerate for long periods of time. We may be given treatments that leave our bodies alive in suspended animation long after the body's intended death. Our bodies may end up being indefinitely hooked to life support equipment without our consent. In a suspended state, we may not be able to communicate our wishes to be let go. This is a frequent issue for families, doctors and hospital administrators as they debate the costs and treatments for *comas, permanent vegetative states* (PVS), or *minimally conscious states* (MCS).

Comas will often be temporary, from a few hours to days, weeks or months. The vegetative and minimally conscious states are typically permanent, however. MCS is accompanied by cognitive ability, while PVS and the coma state leave observers with a question of whether the person is even there. MRI brain scans have illustrated that MCS patients can both recognize speech and respond—if not physically, through their brainwaves. Most coma and PVS patients appear to not be aware of their surroundings at all, however. The difference between a comatose and a PVS patient is simply that the PVS subject appears to be awake. This is deceptive, however, because there is no apparent awareness in the PVS patient. All three states require life support systems—at least feeding tubes—to maintain metabolism. MCS and PVS may only require a feeding tube, while PVS and coma states may also require ventilators.

People do wake up from comas. Waking up from PVS or MCS is rare, however. For this reason, the question of whether to maintain life through artificial means is quite controversial. Since the U.S. court system does not recognize coma, PVS or MCS as death, in the absence of specific instructions by the patient or their legal guardian, the hospital may keep these patients alive indefinitely. It is an ethical question that brings into focus the issues we've discussed here: What is death, and at what point should we let nature take its course?

Note that *euthanasia* or *mercy killing* is not being proposed here. Nor are we condoning suicide in any form, even its slower versions—namely alcoholism and drug abuse. Each of us has a designated time of death according to our consciousness and past behavior. No one has the right to interfere with destiny. This would be fooling around with our most precious asset—

time. Time in itself may not seem precious, but it represents the ability to learn. Every moment we dwell within these bodies is accompanied by needed learning experiences. Even the event of death itself — our leaving the body — is a part of our learning experience.

Each of us can and should make a personal decision of whether we want life support and if so, how long we want to be kept alive with life support should we become comatose, minimally conscious or vegetative. We can decide for ourselves how long life support will be given, if any — and if so, what types of life support treatments are acceptable. We can also predetermine how much pain medication to be given as well. These decisions can be made with or without the duress of pain, as long as we make these decisions while in a state of clarity (again, consult your attorney).

Our health advocate should be easily reachable in the case of our trauma or accident. Our nearest relative is often suggested, but this nearest relative might have some conflict of interest in terms of letting go. Our advocate should approve medications being prescribed according to our wishes. They also can check to make sure those medications match the prescriptions written by the attending physician to avoid hospital errors. Many drug mistakes are made by hospital attendants who misread the doctor's script or mistake one medication for another. The doctor may also not realize a medication allergy exists, and the advocate can clarify this.

The advocate can also monitor whether we are receiving enough fluids and are receiving a good diet during our stay in a hospital or home. Hospitals are notorious for serving overly processed and overly sweetened foods, which can spike our blood sugar and cause a variety of metabolic problems. The advocate may request a special diet for us (hopefully plant-based foods with lots of fiber). They may also consider bringing bottled water, whole foods and supplements to us during their visits to our bedside. The doctor should be made aware of these, however.

Life-support systems may prove valuable in cases where a healthy body has been shot or involved in an accident. However, life-support systems used in enduring efforts to keep elderly people in their bodies past their appointed departure time could very well be classified as cruel and unusual punishment. When it is our time to leave the body, we should be let go without anybody's interference. Natural efforts to restart the heart using the palms or opening the esophagus with the *Heimlich maneuver* may be appropriate. However, the endeavor to put the body on a heart and lung machine or other such invasive methods for a significant duration can merely enslave the inner self to a dysfunctional body.

A visit to the intensive care unit of a local hospital will immediately illustrate this effect. We see unconscious surrogates lying in beds with various tubes and machines running their bodies, like some sort of ghoulish *Cocoon* (1985) scene. Their bodies are doped up, propped up and pumped up with synthetics to keep the blood moving and the brain cells minimally alive. This is not much different from lab scientists keeping cells alive in Petri dishes. The only difference is that leashed to each surrogate body is a trapped inner self likely wanting to move on.

Should we allow the medical institution to manage our healthcare unbridled during critical care, they will generally continue treatment with every possible life-sustaining technology. This is their training. Hospital staff are usually very kind and caring. They may not be trained in the subject matter discussed here, however. Few will have studied ethics or have even read the *Classics*. (The existence of the inner self and the ethical issues of death were profusely discussed in the *Classics* of Aristotle, Socrates, Plato and others.) In addition, hospital staff are typically unaware of the body's absolute need for fresh air, sunlight, clean water and natural foods. Today's critical care institutions are set up to not only bring a body back from its natural death, but to ambulate the body for an indefinite period of time using drugs, life support and restraints. (Yes, most life support patients are strapped into their beds to prevent them from pulling out their life support.)

Our inner self is destined to leave the body at a particular time, determined by a combination of our current state of consciousness (our intentions) and our past activities. Many propose a person's death has been predetermined from birth. Empirical evidence shows that this certainly is not true, however. While a pre-arranged appointment with death might be coded into our body's DNA at birth assuming no further activity, our activities throughout our life in the body alter these projections. Epigenetic research has illustrated that our genetic switches are triggered by our ongoing choices and activities. This is evidenced simply by the many disorders that result from particular lifestyle decisions.

Each of us has a free will as to our intentions. We also have many options on how we exert those intentions as we direct the use of our physical vehicle. The better we care for the body, the longer it will last. This is fundamental to practically any vehicle. If we get regular oil changes and drive with care, our car will likely last longer, for example.

This alone does not guarantee a longer lifespan however. Our time of death is also determined by a complex combination of ongoing intentions and desires, together with the results of our activities and state of consciousness. Our spiritual evolution is something we express directly with pure intention. Should we utilize this lifetime to grow and learn the lessons life presents us with, we will naturally evolve spiritually. This is the Almighty's design for nature's laws of cause and effect.

Our institutions need to support nature's process of aging and dying—and not tease us with denial and futile attempts to avoid death at all costs. We also need to care for the elderly while respecting their experience and knowledge. We need to allow the elderly the ability to ponder the mysteries of existence during their final years without being drugged up and delirious. The world also needs to hear the wisdom of the elderly. The elderly must be able to communicate with the rest of us, to share their lifetime of learning. Stuffing the elderly away in drug-laden institutions is not a good strategy for our society. We need to aid and comfort the elderly without interfering with their mental capacity. Sure, we can provide pain relief. But let's not sacrifice reality for pain relief.

Put quite simply, *old age is not a disease.*

Our Death Bed

The time and circumstances of our departure from this body are critical to our next phase of our journey. Should we be fortunate enough to have some awareness that our body is coming close to death, particular attention should be made to our surroundings and associations during the time of death. Why is this so important?

Our consciousness at the time of death carries us to our next destination. We might compare this to what we might say at the ticket counter at a train station. Should we say "Cleveland," then we'll receive a ticket for a train to Cleveland. We will be in Cleveland before we know it. Should we say "New York," then we'll be traveling to New York City. In any case, what ever is said at that crucial moment at the ticket counter will start the sequences that will drop us at our new destination. This makes the moment we are at the front of the line at the ticket counter extremely important, yes?

We should therefore be as aware as possible during this moment. We should also be surrounded by those who will assist our departure to the right destination, rather than distract us.

Using our analogy, once we made it to the front of the line at the ticket counter at the train station, we would not want to be distracted by a friend who did not understand the importance of buying the right ticket. Perhaps our friend might ask us which apple we want to eat right when we arrive at the ticket counter, so we say to them, *"the big apple."* When the ticket person hears this, we will likely receive a ticket to New York whether we intended to go to New York or not. If we didn't want to go to New York, we might protest receiving the ticket. But since we got what we asked for, we may have to get to the back of the line and wait for some time for a refund and a new ticket. Meanwhile, the train to the destination we wanted to go might leave. All of this because we were not focused on getting the right ticket when it was our turn at the ticket counter. We let someone distract our attention at a critical time.

So what should we be doing at or near our time of death? We should be praying. We should be saying God's Names. We should be thinking of God and our relationship with God. These activities bring our consciousness towards a state of awareness about our intimate relationship with God. As we do this, God and His representatives join us and begin to guide us out of the body. Assuming we have focused at least the more recent part of our lives upon God, He will bring us back home to Him. He will bring us back to that place where we are completely fulfilled: That place where pure love, joy and loving service exist in perfection. This is where each of us come from.

In order to return, we have to be willing to give up our desires to be happy within the physical world. We have to give up desires for wealth, honor, respect, physical beauty, sex and food.

We also have to give up any hatred or jealousy within our hearts. If we are upset about what someone has done to us, we must forgive them and let it go with peace and understanding.

We have to give up our needs to impress others and our desires to be with our family members (although our relationships with them will continue). We have to be willing to give up everything in order to embrace our relationship with God.

While God is a generous, merciful and forgiving Person, and He is our Best Friend, He does require that we dedicate ourselves to Him. He requires that we be willing to give up everything for Him. This is, quite simply, love.

This is no different than many other things in life. In the analogy of the train station, we must be willing to commit to going to New York. We cannot waiver. We cannot say that maybe part of us will go to New York, and part will stay here. We can't send our hands and feet to New York while the rest of our body stays here. That would be ridiculous. We must commit our entire body and mind to the trip in order to get there.

Returning home to Our Best Friend God is no different. We have to commit ourselves to Him. We must be willing to give up everything.

This is made easier when we are leaving our body. When we leave our body, we physically leave everything behind: We leave all our money, all our fame, all our commitments and contracts. We leave everything. The only thing we can take with us is our consciousness. This includes our desires, hopes and dreams. These stay with us and push us into our next destination.

As we should have learned during our physical lifetimes, our own selfish hopes, dreams and desires do not bring us happiness. We are never fulfilled by selfish goals. They may bring fleeting glimpses of fulfillment, but these disappear like sand or water running through our hand when we try to grab them. We are only fulfilled by love for God and His children.

There is scientific proof that our focus upon God brings us to God's presence after death. A number of clinical death experiences have detailed that the patient was brought into God's or His representative's presence after dying. Some reported other angels. In most of these cases, it was communicated to them by God or His representative that it wasn't their time yet: They still had more do to in the physical world. With this communication, they found themselves waking up in their bodies.

Sometimes a person may die in their sleep. Here we may not have the ability to be aware and prepared. What happens in this case? Here the self is mired within the mental body of dreaming as the body dies. In the case, our dream consciousness will determine our direction after death. However, because dreams reflect our desires and consciousness, they are the direct result of how we lived our lives.

If we have lived lives of violence and a struggle to be king of the hill, our dreams will likely contain lots of fighting and struggling. If we die during these dreams, we are likely to take on a body of a violent animal, or an animal subjected to violence.

If we lived our lives focused upon spiritual growth and our relationship with God, our dreams will also reflect this. We will die just as we lived, and our future destination will be determined in kind.

If at some point before our death we release our hopes, dreams and desires to God and completely give ourselves to

Him—trusting that He will guide us and bring us complete ful-fillment—then we will be happy in this life and the next. He will take us into His Arms and completely fulfill us.

How do we get to this place where we are ready to give all our hopes, dreams and desires to God at the time of death? How do we accomplish this consciousness? It takes work and disci-pline. It requires focus prior to the time of death. It is not as if we can live our lives in complete greed with no dedication to God and then right before our time of death we can suddenly change our consciousness.

Our consciousness at the time of death is not determined at death. It is determined over a progressive lifetime within the body. It is determined with each and every decision we make. It is determined by whatever hopes, dreams and desires we have been striving for through our lives. It is this *developed* conscious-ness that will *automatically* arise at the time of death.

This doesn't mean that even up to the time of death we can make changes. We might realize even moments before we leave the body that we were wrong about so much during our lifetime, and we suddenly decide to give our lives to God. This decision can be made at any time. Remember that God is ever-merciful. He is ready to take us back at any time, assuming we are com-mitted to giving ourselves to Him in love.

This is not the same as praying at the last minute because we are afraid of hell. While it is certainly helpful to pray out of fear of going to hell, this does not necessarily achieve the intended destination. It may keep us out of a worse hellish lifetime, how-ever. But because our consciousness is still focused upon our ultimate enjoyment, we are not ready for the spiritual dimen-sion. In this case, we may again take on a human form, where we can keep working towards this goal.

But for those who put off this decision until our body's deathbed, know that there may never be an opportunity for that decision. We may die suddenly in an auto accident. Or we may die in our sleep as discussed.

The time of death can leap upon us at any time. We may not have any time to step back and make the decision to return home. It must be made when there is an opportunity, and that opportunity can come and go quickly.

In other words, the earlier we make this decision the better. The earlier we can decide to give our lives to God (or decide that we will work on giving our lives to God) the more time God will have to train us. The earlier we make the decision to return to God, the more experiences He can give us to prepare for returning home to Him.

Knowing these realities, we can now begin to orient our lives from this moment on to our death bed. We can begin to align our activities to further develop our consciousness towards loving and serving God. We can direct activities in such a way that our lives *remind us* of God at every possible moment. This means that we can pray each day. This means that we can sing God's Names and praise God with every opportunity. This means that we can set up our surroundings to remind us of God.

All of these will awaken our innate consciousness and begin to reveal our intimate relationship with God.

This process continues when we are on our death bed. Should we be fortunate to know our time is coming, we can direct our last hours or minutes. We can invite our spiritual advisor or spiritual peers (of whatever religious discipline we aspire to) into our quarters. In this environment, we can read scripture, pray, say God's Names and sing hymns to God.

As to which of God's Names we choose to sing or pray with, this is up to us. God has many, many authorized Names that have been spread throughout the religious traditions of the world by His loving saints. Whatever theistic discipline we have ascribed to with a tradition that recognizes God as the Supreme Being is acceptable to God. God is not nit-picky. He is not small-minded. He does not give any more attention to a devoted person of Moslem faith than a devoted person of Christian faith, Hindu (monotheistic) faith or any other monotheistic faith.

God does not care what sect or faith we have ascribed to. As long as our focus is upon Him as God—the Supreme Being—He is pleased. As long as our faith is presented to Him single-mindedly with love, respect and humility, He is not disturbed by the specific ritual. This is because God simply wants our love. He doesn't care what tribe, sect, denomination, church or brand of religion we've entertained. In the end it is about our personal relationship with Him that is important.

On the other hand, depending upon the family, having our family members around us at our body's death bed may not be such a good idea. Many family members assume that a person should be with their family as they leave the body. While this can be nice for the person who is not dying, it is not necessarily the best situation for the dying person. Most family members come to see their relatives at their body's deathbed to "pay their respects," but they may have little desire to help send off their relative to the proper destination. Often they are more interested in what they will receive from the estate than they are in the future of the dying person.

At the very least, ones family members will serve to reinforce the concept that we are the body. They are family members because they happen to have received a body in the same family. We know that this is not accidental, however. Two people will typically end up in the same family because they were close friends, married or otherwise intimate in their previous bodies. They end up as family members because of their prior relationship. In other words, friends and family with similar consciousness tend to follow each other from one species and family to the next. This means that our sister may have been our husband in a previous lifetime. Or we may be born within the same dog litter as our current pet dog.

While this might be seen as a warm and cuddly circumstance, it creates an undesirable circumstance of being surrounded by multiple family members at our time of departure from the body. Why? Because as our consciousness is focused upon these people, we will likely continue our physical existence within the 'clan' of this family. We will end up taking on another physical body within whatever species that most of the other clan members will take on or have taken on. If we are fortunate, this might be another human form. But there is also a great likelihood that some of the clan has taken on or will take on bodies of other species. In that case, our focus upon family will dictate that we follow them into that species.

This "herd-like" transmigration from body to body by family members and intimate parties is also driven by consciousness. If our consciousness at the time of death is how much we will miss our family members, we will not be free to go where our spiritual maturity might allow. We will be chained to the destinations of our family members.

This does not mean that our spiritual maturity has no benefit to our family members, however. Should we advance spiritually, and our family members are attached to us, then we can lead them into higher realms after death. As they follow us, they will benefit. But this, of course, will require our spiritual growth prior to the time of death, and the willingness to depart from the clan. If we have had some spiritual advancement yet we are focused upon our family at the time of death, that advancement may be mitigated by their distraction. In other words, perhaps some of the clan headed downwards into the animal kingdom, while another part of the clean resumed human forms. The clan might remain together as some members might be the pets of other human members, for example.

Even a little spiritual advancement can help yield us the human form in our next lifetime. God wants us to continue any advancement we might have accomplished in this lifetime. For this reason, it is urgent that we at least begin to make some progress towards spiritual advancement during the present lifetime. This will assure us of at least continuing our progress as humans or higher species.

On the other hand, perfecting our relationship with God will greatly benefit our family members. Ironically, we can only achieve this if we are willing to give up our family relationships for God. We must be willing to follow Jesus' example, as he said:

> "Who is my mother and who are my brothers? [Pointing to his disciples] Here are my mother and my brothers. For whoever does the will of my Father in heaven is my brother and sister and mother."
> (Matt 12:48-50)

Here Jesus illustrates that our attachment should be upon God, and those who love and serve God. While we can certainly care about our body's family members, we should not be caring about our body's family members in a way that distracts from or depreciates our attachment upon God and our care for others. Every living being is a family member, because we are all children of God. Why should our attention be diverted from our spiritual focus by temporary physical relationships?

If, however, our family members bring to our bedside a focus upon God, this can be a different matter altogether. In such a situation, having family members around our death bed would not necessarily be a distraction, but a benefit, because they would be helping to remind us of our relationship with God.

The best scenario for our death bed is only a few people: perhaps one, two or three people. Optimally, one would be our spiritual advisor of whatever theistic discipline we subscribe to. Another could be a nurse who is ready to assist us in having a drink of water or adjust our bedding. The third can be a person we have been close to through our lives who is willing to read scripture with us or to us, sing God's Names to us, and pray to God with us.

By far the best scenario would be for us to hear God's Names and praises during our departure. God's Names can deliver us to God. Even if we have been selfishly motivated throughout our lifetimes, hearing God's Names at the time of death can provide us with an opportunity to give our lives to Him. It is never too late. This is because God resides within His Names.

If, however, we have no one in the immediate environment who can read scripture, pray with us and/or sing God's Names to us as we are leaving our body, it is better to ask to be left alone so that we can die while focusing upon God. Thus we can sing out or call upon God's Names and read scripture without distraction. We can meditate upon God's beauty and think about how we can one day be with Him. Having privacy during this moment gives us the opportunity for spiritual focus. We won't be distracted by family members or spouses that might be crying over our body and wishing our body would stay with them a few minutes longer. We won't have our heart strings pulled by those who have their own interests at heart. We can let them have their issues, but in another room.

And for those of us who have the opportunity to be at the death bed of our family member or relative, we can consider these issues and consider our contribution. Consider whether we can present prayer and scripture to them at the time of death. Consider whether we can help raise their consciousness during those moments before death by singing God's Names to them or reading scripture.

Should we not have that opportunity at their bedside, or if they lie in a coma, we can step away from their bedside and firmly ask them to be with us for a few moments while we privately pray and/or sing God's Names. We should know that a person in a coma or who has just died (left their body) will almost certainly come around to say goodbye to close family members before they depart. If during this time we are singing God's Names and praying, they will see and hear this. They will have the opportunity to be reminded of God as they are getting ready to release from their physical ties. For many people, as we've learned from clinical death, this may present a moment of clarity for the spiritual self who has just left their body. Hearing God's Names may help guide them towards God at any rate. Even after death a person can have a change of heart.

As for ourselves, we can take comfort in knowing that the death of our body is only a transition. It is not something to fear. We can prepare for that moment with clarity and discipline. We can understand that our body can die at any moment. We can realize that if we train our consciousness for that moment during a time when we do not absolutely need to, we can be prepared for the moment of death. Whether death is five minutes away or fifty years away, there is no difference. We can begin our preparations now, because for each of us, the lessons pertaining to the death of our body may come knocking at any moment.

References and Bibliography

Ackerman D. *A Natural History of the Senses*. New York: Vintage, 1991.

Aissa J, Litime MH, Attis E., Benveniste J. Molecular signalling at high dilution or by means of electronic circuitry. *J Immunol*. 1993;150:A146.

Alexandre P, Darmanyan D, Yushen G, Jenks W, Burel L, Eloy D, Jardon P. Quenching of Singlet Oxygen by Oxygen- and Sulfur-Centered Radicals: Evidence for Energy Transfer to Peroxyl Radicals in Solution. *J. Am. Chem. Soc.*, 120 (2), 396 -403, 1998.

Amassian VE, Cracco RQ, Maccabee PJ. A sense of movement elicited in paralyzed distal arm by focal magnetic coil stimulation of human motor cortex. *Brain Res*. 1989 Feb 13;479(2):355-60.

Ammor MS, Michaelidis C, Nychas GJ. Insights into the role of quorum sensing in food spoilage. *J Food Prot*. 2008 Jul;71(7):1510-25.

Anderson GC, Moore E, Hepworth J, Bergman N. Early skin-to-skin contact for mothers and their healthy newborn infants. *Cochrane Database Syst Rev*. 2003;(2):CD003519.

Appleman P ed. *Darwin: A Norton Critical Edition*. New York: Norton, 1970.

Aronne LJ, Thornton-Jones ZD. New targets for obesity pharmacotherapy. *Clin Pharmacol Ther*. 2007 May;81(5):748-52.

Asimov I. *The Chemicals of Life*. New York: Signet, 1954.

Askeland D. *The Science and Engineering of Materials*. Boston: PWS, 1994.

Aspect A, Grangier P, Roger G. Experimental Realization of Einstein-Podolsky-Rosen-Bohm Gedankenexperiment: A New Violation of Bell's Inequalities. *Physical Review Letters*. 1982;49(2): 91-94.

Aton SJ, Colwell CS, Harmar AJ, Waschek J, Herzog ED. Vasoactive intestinal polypeptide mediates circadian rhythmicity and synchrony in mammalian clock neurons. *Nat Neurosci*. 2005 Apr;8(4):476-83.

Avanzini G, Lopez L, Koelsch S, Majno M. The Neurosciences and Music II: From Perception to Performance. *Annals of the New York Academy of Sciences*. 2006 Mar;1060.

Aymard JP, Aymard B, Netter P, Bannwarth B, Trechot P, Streiff F. Haematological adverse effects of histamine H2-receptor antagonists. *Med Toxicol Adverse Drug Exp*. 1988 Nov-Dec;3(6):430-48.

Bach E. *Heal Thyself*. Saffron Walden: CW Daniel, 1931-2003.

Bache C. *Lifecycles: Reincarnation and the Web of Life*. New York: Paragon House, 1994.

Backster C. *Primary Perception: Biocommunication with Plants, Living Foods, and Human Cells*. Anza, CA: White Rose Millennium Press, 2003.

Bader J. The relative power of SNPs and haplotype as genetic markers for association tests. *Pharmacogenomics*. 2001;2:11-24.

Bai H, Yu P, Yu M. Effect of electroacununcture on sex hormone levels in patients with Sjogren's syndrome. *Zhen Ci Yan Jiu*. 2007;32(3):203-6.

Baker DW. An introduction to the theory and practice of German electroacupuncture and accompanying medications. *Am J Acupunct*. 1984;12:327-332.

Ballentine RM. *Radical Healing*. New York: Harmony Books, 1999.

Bannerjee H. *Americans Who Have Been Reincarnated*. New York: Macmillan, 1980.

Banyo T. The role of electrical neuromodulation in the therapy of chronic lower urinary tract dysfunction. *Ideggyogy Sz*. 2003 Jan 20;56(1-2):68-71.

Baranauskas G, Nistri A. Sensitization of pain pathways in the spinal cord: cellular mechanisms. *Prog Neurobiol*. 1998 Feb;54(3):349-65.

Barber CF. The use of music and colour theory as a behaviour modifier. *Br J Nurs*. 1999 Apr 8-21;8(7):443-8.

Barker A. *Scientific Method in Ptolemy's Harmonics*. Cambridge: Cambridge University Press, 2000.

Barron M. Light exposure, melatonin secretion, and menstrual cycle parameters: an integrative review. *Biol Res Nurs*. 2007 Jul;9(1):49-69.

Bastide M, Doucet-Jaboeuf M, Daurat V. Activity and chronopharmacology of very low doses of physiological immune inducers. *Immun Today*. 1985;6: 234-235.

Bastide M. Immunological examples on ultra high dilution research. In: Endler P, Schulte J (eds.): *Ultra High Dilution. Physiology and Physics*. Dordrech: Kluwer Academic Publishers, 1994:27-34.

Bates DW, Cullen DJ, Laird N, Petersen LA, Small SD, Servi D, Laffel G, Sweitzer BJ, Shea BF, Hallisey R, *et al*. Incidence of adverse drug events and potential adverse drug events. Implications for prevention. ADE Prevention Study Group. *JAMA*. 1995 Jul 5;274(1):29-34.

Becker R. *Cross Currents*. Los Angeles: Jeremy P. Tarcher, 1990.

Becker R. *The Body Electric*. New York: William Morrow, 1985.

Beckerman H, Becher J, Lankhorst GJ. The effectiveness of vibratory stimulation in anejaculatory men with spinal cord injury. *Paraplegia*. 1993 Nov;31(11):689-99.

Beeson, C. The moon and plant growth. *Nature*. 1946;158:572-3.

Bell B, Defouw R. Concerning a lunar modulation of geomagnetic activity. *J Geophys Res*. 1964;69:3169-3174.

Beloff J. Parapsychology and radical dualism. *J Rel & Psych Res*. 1985;8, 3-10.

Benedetti F, Radaelli D, Bernasconi A, Dallaspezia S, Falini A, Scotti G, Lorenzi C, Colombo C, Smeraldi E. Clock genes beyond the clock: CLOCK genotype biases neural correlates of moral valence decision in depressed patients. *Genes Brain Behav*. 2007 Mar 26.

Bennett GJ, Update on the neurophysiology of pain transmission and modulation: focus on the NMDA-receptor. *J Pain Symptom Manage*. 2000;19 (suppl 1):S.:2-6.

Benor D. Healing Research. Volume 1. Munich, Germany: Helix Verlag, 1992.

Bentley E. *Awareness: Biorhythms, Sleep and Dreaming*. London: Routledge, 2000

Benveniste J, Aïssa J, Guillonnet D. A simple and fast method for in vivo demonstration of electromagnetic molecular signaling (EMS) via high dilution or computer recording. *FASEB Jnl*. 1999;13: A163.

Benveniste J, Aïssa J, Guillonnet D. Digital Biology : Specificity of the digitized molecular signal. *FASEB Jnl*. 1998;12: A412.

Benveniste J, Aïssa J, Litime M, Tsangaris G, Thomas Y. Transfer of the molecular signal by electronic amplification. *FASEB J*. 1994;8:A398.

Berk M, Dodd S, Henry M. Do ambient electromagnetic fields affect behaviour? A demonstration of the relationship between geomagnetic storm activity and suicide. *Bioelectromagnetics*. 2006 Feb;27(2):151-5.

Bertin G. *Spiral Structure in Galaxies: A Density Wave Theory*. Cambridge: MIT Press, 1996.

Bishop B. Pain: its physiology and rationale for management. Part III. Consequences of current concepts of pain mechanisms related to pain management. *Phys Ther*. 1980 Jan;60(1):24-37.

Bishop, C. Moon influence in lettuce growth. *Astrol J*. 1977;10(1):13-15.

Bitbol M, Luisi PL. Autopoiesis with or without cognition: defining life at its edge. *J R Soc Interface*. 2004 Nov 22;1(1):99-107.

Blackmore SJ. Near-death experiences. *J R Soc Med*. 1996 Feb;89(2):73-6.

Bockemühl, J. *Towards a Phenomenology of the Etheric World*. New York: Anthroposophical Press, 1985.

Bodnar L, Simhan H. The prevalence of preterm birth varies by season of last menstrual period. *Am J Obst and Gyn*. 2003:195(6);S211-S211.

Boivin DB, Czeisler CA. Resetting of circadian melatonin and cortisol rhythms in humans by ordinary room light. *Neuroreport*. 1998 Mar 30;9(5):779-82.

Boivin DB, Duffy JF, Kronauer RE, Czeisler CA. Dose-response relationships for resetting of human circadian clock by light. *Nature*. 1996 Feb 8;379(6565):540-2.

Bose J. *Response in the Living and Non-Living*. New York: Longmans, Green & Co., 1902.

Bottorff JL. The use and meaning of touch in caring for patients with cancer. *Oncol Nurs Forum*. 1993 Nov-Dec;20(10):1531-8.

Bourgine P, Stewart J. Autopoiesis and cognition. *Artif Life*. 2004 Summer;10(3):327-45.

Bowler PJ. *The Eclipse of Darwinism: Antievolutionary Theories in the Decades Around 1900*. Baltimore: Johns Hopkins, 1983.

Brasseur JG, Nicosia MA, Pal A, Miller LS. Function of longitudinal vs circular muscle fibers in esophageal peristalsis, deduced with mathematical modeling. *World J Gastroenterol*. 2007 Mar 7;13(9):1335-46.

REFERENCES AND BIBLIOGRAPHY

Braude S. *First Person Plural: Multiple Personality and the Philosophy of Mind.* Landham, MD: Rowman & Littlefield, 1995.

Britton WB, Bootzin RR. Near-death experiences and the temporal lobe. *Psychol Sci.* 2004 Apr;15(4):254-8.

Brodeur P. *Currents of Death.* New York: Simon and Schuster, 1989.

Brown V. *The Amateur Naturalists Handbook.* Englewood Cliffs, NJ: Prentice-Hall, 1980.

Brown, F. The rhythmic nature of animals and plants. *Cycles.* 1960 Apr:81-92.

Brown, J. Stimulation-produced analgesia: acupuncture, TENS and alternative techniques. *Anaesthesia &intensive care medicine.* 2005 Feb;6(2):45-47.

Browne J. Developmental Care - Considerations for Touch and Massage in the Neonatal Intensive Care Unit. *Neonatatal Network.* 2000 Feb;19(1).

Buck L, Axel R. A novel multigene family may encode odorant receptors: A molecule basis for odor recognition. *Cell.* 1991;65(April 5):175-187.

Buijs RM, Scheer FA, Kreier F, Yi C, Bos N, Goncharuk VD, Kalsbeek A. Organization of circadian functions: interaction with the body. *Prog Brain Res.* 2006;153:341-60.

Bulsing PJ, Smeets MA, van den Hout MA. Positive Implicit Attitudes toward Odor Words. *Chem Senses.* 2007 May 7.

Burnham K, Andersson D. *Model Selection and Inference. A Practical Information-Theoretic Approach.* New York: Springer, 1998

Burr H, Hovland C. Bio-Electric Potential Gradients in the Chick. *Yale Journal of Biology & Medicine.* 1937;9:247-258

Burr H, Lane C, Nims L. A Vacuum Tube Microvoltmeter for the Measurement of Bioelectric Phenomena. *Yale Journal of Biology & Medicine.* 1936;10:65-76.

Burr H, Smith G, Strong L. Bio-electric Properties of Cancer-Resistant and Cancer-Susceptible Mice. *American Journal of Cancer.* 1938;32:240-248

Burr H. *The Fields of Life.* New York: Ballantine, 1972.

Buzsaki G. Theta rhythm of navigation: link between path integration and landmark navigation, episodic and semantic memory. *Hippocampus.* 2005;15(7):827-40.

Calvin W. *The Handbook of Brain Theory and Neural Networks.* Boston: MIT Press, 1995.

Campbell A. The role of aluminum and copper on neuroinflammation and Alzheimer's disease. *J Alzheimers Dis.* 2006 Nov;10(2-3):165-72.

Capitani D, Yethiraj A, Burnell EE. Memory effects across surfactant mesophases. *Langmuir.* 2007 Mar 13;23(6):3036-48.

Cassileth B, Trevisan C, Gubili J. Complementary therapies for cancer pain. *Curr Pain Headache Rep.* 2007 Aug;11(4):265-9.

Cavalli-Sforza L, Feldman M. *Cultural Transmission and Evolution: A quantitative approach.* Princeton: Princeton UP, 1981.

Cengel YA, *Heat Transfer: A Practical Approach.* Boston: McGraw-Hill, 1998.

Chaitow L. *Conquer Pain the Natural Way.* San Francisco: Chronicle Books, 2002.

Choi DW. Glutamate neurotoxicity and diseases of the nervous system. *Neuron.* 1988;1:623-34.

Churchill G, Doerge R. Empirical threshold values for quantitative trait mapping. *Genetics* 1994;138:963-971.

Chwirot WB, Popp F. White-light-induced luminescence and mitotic activity of yeast cells. *Folia Histochemica et Cytobiologica.* 1991;29(4):155.

Citro M, Endler PC, Pongratz W, Vinattieri C, Smith CW, Schulte J. Hormone effects by electronic transmission. *FASEB J.* 1995:Abstract 12161.

Citro M, Smith CW, Scott-Morley A, Pongratz W, Endler PC. Transfer of information from molecules by means of electronic amplification, in P.C. Endler, J. Schulte (eds.): *Ultra High Dilution. Physiology and Physics.* Dordrecht: Kluwer Academic Publishers. 1994;209-214.

Cocilovo A. Colored light therapy: overview of its history, theory, recent developments and clinical applications combined with acupuncture. *Am J Acupunct.* 1999;27(1-2):71-83.

Cohen S, Popp F. Biophoton emission of the human body. *J Photochem & Photobio.* 1997;B 40:187-189.

Cohen S, Popp F. Low-level luminescence of the human skin. *Skin Res Tech.* 1997;3:177-180.

Conely J. Music and the Military. *Air University Review.* 1972 Mar-Ap.

Contreras D, Steriade M. Cellular basis of EEG slow rhythms: a study of dynamic corticothalamic relationships. *J Neurosci*. 1995 Jan;15(1 Pt 2):604-22.

Cook J, The Therapeutic Use of Music. *Nursing Forum*. 1981;20:3: 253-66.

Corkin S, Amaral DG, González RG, et al: H. M.'s medial temporal lobe lesion: findings from magnetic resonance imaging. *J Neurosci*. 1997;17:3964-3979.

Cox CB. Emory-led Study Links Metals to Alzheimer's and Other Neurodegenerative Diseases. *Emory Univ Mag*. 2007 Aug 10.

Craciunescu CN, Wu R, Zeisel SH. Diethanolamine alters neurogenesis and induces apoptosis in fetal mouse hippocampus. *FASEB J*. 2006 Aug;20(10):1635-40.

Crick F. *Life Itself: Its Origin and Nature*. New York: Simon and Schuster, 1981.

Crofford LJ. Neuroendocrine abnormalities in fibromyalgia and related disorders. *Am J Med Sci*. 1998;315:359-66.

Cross ML. Immune-signalling by orally-delivered probiotic bacteria: effects on common mucosal immunoresponses and protection at distal mucosal sites. Int J Immunopathol Pharmacol. 2004 May-Aug;17(2):127-134.

Cruccu G, Aziz TZ, Garcia-Larrea L, Hansson P, Jensen TS, Lefaucheur JP, Simpson BA, Taylor RS. EFNS guidelines on neurostimulation therapy for neuropathic pain. *Eur J Neurol*. 2007 Sep;14(9):952-70.

Cummings M. *Human Heredity: Principles and Issues*. St. Paul, MN: West, 1988.

Curtis LH, Østbye T, Sendersky V, Hutchison S, Dans PE, Wright A, Woosley RL, Schulman KA. Inappropriate prescribing for elderly Americans in a large outpatient population. *Arch Intern Med*. 2004 Aug 9-23;164(15):1621-5.

Cuthbert SC, Goodheart GJ Jr. On the reliability and validity of manual muscle testing: a literature review. *Chiropr Osteopat*. 2007 Mar 6;15:4.

Dalmose A, Bjarkam C, Vuckovic A, Sorensen JC, Hansen J. Electrostimulation: a future treatment option for patients with neurogenic urodynamic disorders? *APMIS Suppl*. 2003;(109):45-51.

Darrow K. *The Renaissance of Physics*. New York: Macmillan, 1936.

DaVinci L. (Dickens E. ed.) *The Da Vinci Notebooks*. London: Profile, 2005.

Dawkins R. *Climbing Mount Improbable*. New York: Viking Press, 1996.

Dawkins R. *River out of Eden*. London: Weidenfeld and Nicholson, 1995.

Dawkins R. *The Blind Watchmaker*. Essex: Longman Scientific and Technical, 1986.

Dawkins R. *The Selfish Gene*. Oxford: Oxford UP, 1977 (1989 edition).

Dean C. *Death by Modern Medicine*. Belleville, ON: Matrix Verite-Media, 2005.

Dean E, Mihalasky J, Ostrander S, Schroeder L. *Executive ESP*. Englewood Cliffs, NJ: Prentice-Hall, 1974.

Dean E. Infrared measurements of healer-treated water. In: Roll W, Beloff J, White R (Eds.): *Research in parapsychology 1982*. Metuchen, NJ: Scarecrow Press, 1983:100-101.

Defrin R, Ohry A, Blumen N, Urca G. Sensory determinants of thermal pain. *Brain*. 2002 Mar;125(Pt 3):501-10.

Deitel M. Applications of electrical pacing in the body. *Obes Surg*. 2004 Sep;14 Suppl 1:S3-8.

Delcomyn F. *Foundations of Neurobiology*. New York: W.H. Freeman and Co., 1998.

Dement W, Vaughan C. *The Promise of Sleep*. New York: Dell, 1999.

Dennett D. *Brainstorms: Philosophical Essays on Mind & Psychology*. Cambridge: MIT Press., 1980.

Dennett D. *Consciousness Explained*. London: Little, Brown and Co., 1991.

Depue BE, Banich MT, Curran T. Suppression of emotional and nonemotional content in memory: effects of repetition on cognitive control. *Psychol Sci*. 2006 May;17(5):441-7.

Dere E, Kart-Teke E, Huston JP, De Souza Silva MA. The case for episodic memory in animals. *Neurosci Biobehav Rev*. 2006;30(8):1206-24.

Devulder J, Crombez E, Mortier E. Central pain: an overview. *Acta Neurol Belg*. 2002 Sep;102(3):97-103.

Dhond RP, Kettner N, Napadow V. Neuroimaging acupuncture effects in the human brain. *J Altern Complement Med*. 2007 Jul-Aug;13(6):603-16.

Dieter JN, Field T, Hernandez-Reif M, Emory EK, Redzepi M. Stable preterm infants gain more weight and sleep less after five days of massage therapy. *J Pediatr Psychol.* 2003 Sep;28(6):403-11.

Dimitriadis GD, Raptis SA. Thyroid hormone excess and glucose intolerance. *Exp Clin Endocrinol Diabetes.* 2001;109 Suppl 2:S225-39.

Dobrowolski J, Ezzahir A, Knapik M. Possibilities of chemiluminescence application in comparative studies of animal and cancer cells with special attention to leucemic blood cells. In: Jezowska-Trzebiatowska, B., *et al.* (eds.). *Photon Emission from Biological Systems.* Singapore: World Scientific Publ, 1987:170-183.

Dolcos F, LaBar KS, Cabeza R. Interaction between the amygdala and the medial temporal lobe memory system predicts better memory for emotional events. *Neuron.* 2004 Jun 10;42(5):855-63.

Duke M. *Acupuncture.* New York: Pyramid, 1973.

Dunlop KA, Carson DJ, Shields MD. Hypoglycemia due to adrenal suppression secondary to high-dose nebulized corticosteroid. *Pediatr Pulmonol.* 2002 Jul;34(1):85-6.

Dunne B, Jahn R, Nelson R. Precognitive Remote Perception. Princeton Engineering Anomalies *Res Lab Rep.* Princeton. 1983 Aug.

Eden D, Feinstein D. *Energy Medicine.* New York: Penguin Putnam, 1998.

Edwards B. *Drawing on the Right Side of the Brain.* Los Angeles, CA: Tarcher, 1979.

Edwards R, Ibison M, Jessel-Kenyon J, Taylor R. Light emission from the human body. *Comple Med Res.* 1989;3(2): 16-19.

Edwards R, Ibison M, Jessel-Kenyon J, Taylor R. Measurements of human bioluminescence. *Acup Elect Res, Intl Jnl,* 1990;15: 85-94.

Edwards, L. *The Vortex of Life, Nature's Patterns in Space and Time.* Floris Press, 1993.

Egon G, Chartier-Kastler E, Denys P, Ruffion A. Spinal cord injury patient and Brindley neurostimulation. *Prog Urol.* 2007 May;17(3):535-9.

Electromagnetic fields: the biological evidence. *Science.* 1990;249: 1378-1381.

Electronic Evidence of Auras, Chakras in UCLA Study. *Brain/Mind Bulletin.* 1978;3:9 Mar 20.

Ellison CG, Burdette AM, Hill TD. Blessed assurance: religion, anxiety, and tranquility among US adults. *Soc Sci Res.* 2009 Sep;38(3):656-67.

Erdelyi R. MHD waves and oscillations in the solar plasma. Introduction. *Philos Transact A Math Phys Eng Sci.* 2006 Feb 15;364(1839):289-96.

Esch T, Stefano GB. The Neurobiology of Love. *Neuro Endocrinol Lett.* 2005 Jun;26(3):175-92.

Evans P, Forte D, Jacobs C, Fredhoi C, Aitchison E, Hucklebridge F, Clow A. Cortisol secretory activity in older people in relation to positive and negative well-being. *Psychoneuroendocrinology.* 2007 Aug 7

Falcon CT. *Happiness and Personal Problems.* Lafayette, LA: Sensible Psychology, 1992.

Field TM, Schanberg SM, Scafidi F, Bauer CR, Vega-Lahr N, Garcia R, Nystrom J, Kuhn CM. Tactile/kinesthetic stimulation effects on preterm neonates. *Pediatrics.* 1986 May;77(5):654-8.

Forget-Dubois N, Boivin M, Dionne G, Pierce T, Tremblay RE, Perusse D. A longitudinal twin study of the genetic and environmental etiology of maternal hostile-reactive behavior during infancy and toddlerhood. *Infant Behav Dev.* 2007 Aug;30(3):453-65.

Frawley D, Lad V. *The Yoga of Herbs.* Sante Fe: Lotus Press, 1986.

Freeman W. *The Physiology of Perception. Sci. Am.* 1991 Feb.

Frey A. Electromagnetic field interactions with biological systems. *FASEB Jnl.* 1993;7: 272-28.

Fucile S, Gisel EG, Lau C. Effect of an oral stimulation program on sucking skill maturation of preterm infants. *Dev Med Child Neurol.* 2005 Mar;47(3):158-62.

Fukumoto H, Tokuda T, Kasai T, Ishigami N, Hidaka H, Kondo M, Allsop D, Nakagawa M. High-molecular-weight {beta}-amyloid oligomers are elevated in cerebrospinal fluid of Alzheimer patients. *FASEB J.* 2010 Mar 25.

Fuster JM. Prefrontal neurons in networks of executive memory. *Brain Res Bull.* 2000 Jul 15;52(5):331-6.

Gabriel S, Schaffner S, Nguyen H, Moore J, Roy J. The structure of haplotype blocks in the human genome. *Science.* 2002;296:2225-2229.

Galaev, YM. The Measuring of Ether-Drift Velocity and Kinematic Ether Viscosity within Optical Wave Bands. *Spacetime & Substance*. 2002;3(5): 207-224.

Gambini JP, Velluti RA, Pedemonte M. Hippocampal theta rhythm synchronizes visual neurons in sleep and waking. *Brain Res*. 2002 Feb 1;926(1-2):137-41.

Gandhi T, Weingart S, Borus J, Seger A, Peterson J, Burdick E, Seger D, Shu K, Federico F, Leape L, Bates D. Adverse drug events in ambulatory care. *N Engl J Med*. 2003 Apr 17;348(16):1556-64.

Garcia-Lazaro JA, Ahmed B, Schnupp JW. Tuning to natural stimulus dynamics in primary auditory cortex. *Curr Biol*. 2006 Feb 7;16(3):264-71.

Gau SS, Soong WT, Merikangas KR. Correlates of sleep-wake patterns among children and young adolescents in Taiwan. *Sleep*. 2004 May 1;27(3):512-9.

Gerber R. *Vibrational Healing*. Sante Fe: Bear, 1988.

Gisler GC, Diaz J, Duran N. Observations on Blood Plasma Chemiluminescence in Normal Subjects and Cancer Patients. *Arq Biol Tecnol*. 1983;26(3):345-352.

Glover J. *The Philosophy of Mind*. Oxford University Press, 1976.

Goldberg B. *Past Lives, Future Lives*. New York: Ballantine, 1982.

Golub E. *The Limits of Medicine*. New York: Times Books, 1994.

Gomez-Abellan P, Hernandez-Morante JJ, Lujan JA, Madrid JA, Garaulet M. Clock genes are implicated in the human metabolic syndrome. *Int J Obes*. 2007 Jul 24.

Gould SJ. *Eight Little Piggies*. New York: Norton, 1993.

Gould SJ. *Wonderful Life: The Burgess Shale and the nature of history*. New York: Penguin Books, 1989.

Grad B, Dean E. Independent confirmation of infrared healer effects. In: White R, Broughton R (Eds.): *Research in parapsychology 1983*. Metuchen, NJ: Scarecrow Press, 1984:81-83.

Grad B. A Telekinetic Effect on Plant Growth. *Intl Jnl Parapsy*. 1964;6: 473.

Grad B. The 'Laying on of Hands': Implications for Psychotherapy, Gentling, and the Placebo Effect. *Jnl Amer Soc for Psych Res*. 1967 Oct;61(4): 286-305.

Grad, B. A telekinetic effect on plant growth: II. Experiments involving treatment of saline in stoppered bottles. *Internl J Parapsychol*. 1964;6:473-478, 484-488.

Grasmuller S, Irnich D. Acupuncture in pain therapy. *MMW Fortschr Med*. 2007 Jun 21;149(25-26):37-9.

Grasso F, Musumeci F, Triglia A, Rodolico G, Cammisuli F, Rinzivillo C, Fragati G, Santuccio A, Rodolico M. In Stanley P, Kricka L (ed). *Ultraweak Luminescence from Cancer Tissues. In Bioluminescence and Chemiluminescence - Current Status*. New York: J Wiley & Sons. 1991:277-280.

Grasso F, Musumeci F, Triglia A. Yanbastiev M. Borisova, S. Self-irradiation effect on yeast cells. *Photochemistry and Photobiology*. 1991;54(1):147-149.

Grissom C. Magnetic field effects in biology: A survey of possible mechanisms with emphasis on radical pair recombination. *Chem. Rev*. 1995;95: 3-24.

Grobstein P. Directed movement in the frog: motor choice, spatial representation, free will? *Neurobiology of motor programme selection*. Pergamon Press, 1992.

Gupta A, Rash GS, Somia NN, Wachowiak MP, Jones J, Desoky A. The motion path of the digits. *J Hand Surg*. 1998; 23A:1038-1042.

Hagins WA, Penn RD, Yoshikami S. Dark current and photocurrent in retinal rods. *Biophys J*. 1970 May;10(5):380-412.

Hagins WA, Robinson WE, Yoshikami S. Ionic aspects of excitation in rod outer segments. *Ciba Found Symp*. 1975;(31):169-89.

Hagins WA, Yoshikami S. Ionic mechanisms in excitation of photoreceptors. *Ann N Y Acad Sci*. 1975 Dec 30;264:314-25.

Hagins WA, Yoshikami S. Proceedings: A role for Ca2+ in excitation of retinal rods and cones. *Exp Eye Res*. 1974 Mar;18(3):299-305.

Hagins WA. The visual process: Excitatory mechanisms in the primary receptor cells. *Annu Rev Biophys Bioeng*. 1972;1:131-58.

Halliday GM, Agar NS, Barnetson RS, Ananthaswamy HN, Jones AM. UV-A fingerprint mutations in human skin cancer. *Photochem Photobiol*. 2005 Jan-Feb;81(1):3-8.

Halpern S. *Tuning the Human Instrument*. Palo Alto, CA: Spectrum Research Institute, 1978.

Hamel P. *Through Music to the Self: How to Appreciate and Experience Music*. Boulder: Shambala, 1979.

Hameroff SR, Penrose R. Conscious events as orchestrated spacetime selections. *J Consc Studies*. 1996;3(1):36-53.

Hameroff SR, Penrose R. Orchestrated reduction of quantum coherence in brain microtubules: A model for consciousness. In: Hameroff SN, Kaszniak A, Scott AC (eds.): *Toward a Science of Consciousness - The First Tucson Discussions and Debates*. Cambridge: MIT Press, 1996.

Hameroff SR, Smith, S, Watt.R. Nonlinear electrodynamics in cytoskeletal protein lattices. In: Adey W, Lawrence A (eds.), *Nonlinear Electrodynamics in Biological Systems*. 1984:567-583.

Hameroff SR, Watt, R. Information processing in microtubules. *J Theor Biology*. 1982;98:549-561.

Hameroff SR. Coherence in the cytoskeleton: Implications for biological information processing. In: Fröhlich H. (ed.): *Biological Coherence and Response to External Stimuli*. Springer, Berlin-New York 1988, pp.242-264.

Hameroff SR. Light is heavy: Wave mechanics in proteins - A microtubule hologram model of consciousness. *Proceedings 2nd. International Congress on Psychotronic Research*. Monte Carlo, 1975:168-169.

Hameroff SR. The "conscious pilot"-dendritic synchrony moves through the brain to mediate consciousness. *J Biol Phys*. 2010 Jan;36(1):71-93.

Hameroff SR. *Ultimate Biocomputing - Biomolecular Consciousness and Nanotechnology*. Amsterdam: Elsevier, 1987.

Hameroff, SR. Ch'i: A neural hologram? Microtubules, bioholography and acupuncture. *Am J Chin Med*. 1974;2(2):163-170.

Hans J. *The Structure and Dynamics of Waves and Vibrations*. New York:.Schocken and Co., 1975.

Harlow HF, Dodsworth RO, Harlow MK. Total social isolation in monkeys. *Proc Natl Acad Sci U S A*. 1965.

Harlow HF. Development of affection in primates. In Bliss E (ed): *Roots of Behavior*. New York: Harper, 1962: 157-166.

Harlow HF. Early social deprivation and later behavior in the monkey. In: Abrams A, Gurner H, Tomal J (eds): *Unfinished tasks in the behavioral sciences*. Baltimore: Williams & Wilkins. 1964: 154-173.

Hayes JA. TAC-TIC therapy: a non-pharmacological stroking intervention for premature infants. *Complement Ther Nurs Midwifery*. 1998 Feb;4(1):25-7.

Heinrich H. Assessment of non-sinusoidal, pulsed, or intermittent exposure to low frequency electric and magnetic fields. *Health Phys*. 2007 Jun;92(6):541-6.

Helms JA, Farnham PJ, Segal E, Chang HY. Functional demarcation of active and silent chromatin domains in human HOX loci by noncoding RNAs. *Cell*. 2007 Jun 29;129(7):1311-23.

Hernandez-Reif M, Diego M, Field T. Preterm infants show reduced stress behaviors and activity after 5 days of massage therapy. *Infant Behav Dev*. 2007 Dec;30(4):557-61.

Heyers D, Manns M, Luksch H, Gu¨ntu¨ rku¨n O, Mouritsen H. A Visual Pathway Links Brain Structures Active during Magnetic Compass Orientation in Migratory Birds. *PLoS One*. 2007;2(9): e937. 2007.

Hillecke T, Nickel A, Bolay HV. Scientific perspectives on music therapy. *Ann N Y Acad Sci*. 2005 Dec;1060:271-82.

Hobbs C. *Stress & Natural Healing*. Loveland, CO: Interweave Press, 1997.

Hollwich F. Hartmann C. Influence of light through the eyes on metabolism and hormones. *Ophtalmologie*. 1990;4(4):385-9.

Hollwich F. *The influence of ocular light perception on metabolism in man and in animal*. New York: Springer-Verlag, 1979.

Holmquist G. Susumo Ohno left us January 13, 2000, at the age of 71. *Cytogenet and Cell Genet*. 2000;88:171-172.

Hope M. *The Psychology of Healing*. Longmead UK: Element Books, 1989.

Hoskin M.(ed.). *The Cambridge Illustrated History of Astronomy*. Cambridge: Cambridge Press, 1997.

Hoyle F. *Evolution from Space*. Londong: JM Dent, 1981.

Huffman C. Archytas of Tarentum: *Pythagorean, philosopher and Mathematician King*. Cambridge: Cambridge University Press, 2005.

Hull D. *Science as a Process: An evolutionary account of the social and conceptual development of science*. Chicago: Univ Chicago Press, 1988.

Hunt V. *Infinite Mind: Science of the Human Vibrations of Consciousness*. Malibu: Malibu Publ. 2000.

Hur YM, Rushton JP. Genetic and environmental contributions to prosocial behaviour in 2- to 9-year-old South Korean twins. *Biol Lett*. 2007 Aug 28.

Inaba H. INABA Biophoton. Exploratory Research for Advanced Technology. *Japan Science and Technology Agency*. 1991. http://www.jst.go.jp/erato/project/isf_P/isf_P.html. Acc. 2006 Nov.

International HapMap Consortium. The international HapMap project. *Nature*. 2003;426:789-794.

Jahn R, Dunne, B. *Margins of Reality: the Role of Consciousness in the Physical World*. New York: Harcourt Brace Jovanovich, 1987.

Janssens D, Delaive E, Houbion A, Eliaers F, Remacle J, Michiels C. Effect of venotropic drugs on the respiratory activity of isolated mitochondria and in endothelial cells. *Br J Pharmacol*. 2000 Aug;130(7):1513-24.

Jensen HK. The molecular genetic basis and diagnosis of familial hypercholesterolemia in Denmark. *Dan Med Bull*. 2002 Nov;49(4):318-45.

Ji Y, Liu YB, Zheng LY, Zhang XQ. Survey of studies on tissue structures and biological characteristics of channel lines. *Zhongguo Zhen Jiu*. 2007 Jun;27(6):427-32.

Johari H. *Ayurvedic Massage: Traditional Indian Techniques for Balancing Body and Mind*. Rochester, VT: Healing Arts, 1996.

Johari H. *Chakras*. Rochester, VT: Destiny, 1987.

Johnston A. A spatial property of the retino-cortical mapping. *Spatial Vision*. 1986;1(4):319-331.

Johnston RE. Pheromones, the vomeronasal system, and communication. From hormonal responses to individual recognition. *Ann N Y Acad Sci*. 1998 Nov 30;855:333-48.

Kandel E, Siegelbaum S, Schwartz J. *Synaptic transmission. Principles of Neural Science*. New York: Elsevier, 1991.

Karis TE, Jhon MS. Flow-induced anisotropy in the susceptibility of a particle suspension. *Proc Natl Acad Sci USA*. 1986 Jul;83(14):4973-4977.

Karnstedt J. Ions and Consciousness. *Whole Self*. 1991 Spring.

Keil J, Stevenson I. Do cases of the reincarnation type show similar features over many years? A study of Turkish cases. *J. Sci. Exploration*. 1999;13(2) 189-198.

Keil J. New cases in Burma, Thailand, and Turkey: A limited field study replication of some aspects of Ian Stevenson's work. *J. Sci. Exploration*. 1991;5(1):27-59.

Kelder P. *Ancient Secret of the Fountain of Youth: Book 1*. New York: Doubleday, 1998.

Kerr CC, Rennie CJ, Robinson PA. Physiology-based modeling of cortical auditory evoked potentials. *Biol Cybern*. 2008 Feb;98(2):171-84.

Key T, Appleby P, Davey G, Allen N, Spencer E, Travis R. Mortality in British vegetarians: review and preliminary results from EPIC-Oxford. *Amer. Jour. Clin. Nutr. Suppl*. 2003;78(3): 533S-538S.

Kiecolt-Glaser JK, Graham JE, Malarkey WB, Porter K, Lemeshow S, Glaser R. Olfactory influences on mood and autonomic, endocrine, and immune function. *Psychoneuroendocrinology*. 2008 Apr;33(3):328-39.

Kirlian SD, Kirlian V, Photography and Visual Observation by Means of High-Frequency Currents. *J Sci Appl Photog*. 1963;6(6).

Klaus M. Mother and infant: early emotional ties. *Pediatrics*. 1998 Nov;102(5 Suppl E):1244-6.

Klein E, Smith D, Laxminarayan R. Trends in Hospitalizations and Deaths in the United States Associated with Infections Caused by *Staphylococcus aureus* and MRSA, 1999-2004. *Emerging Infectious Diseases*. University of Florida Press Release. 2007 Dec 3.

Klein R, Landau MG. *Healing: The Body Betrayed*. Minneapolis: DCI:Chronimed, 1992.

Klima H, Haas O, Roschger P. Photon emission from blood cells and its possible role in immune system regulation. In: Jezowska-Trzebiatowska B., *et al.* (eds.): *Photon Emission from Biological Systems*. Singapore: World Scientific, 1987:153-169.

Kloss J. *Back to Eden*. Twin Oaks, WI: Lotus Press, 1939-1999.

Koch C. Debunking the Digital Brain. *Sci. Am.* 1997 Feb.

Koszowski B, Goniewicz M, Czogala J. Alternative methods of nicotine dependence treatment. *Przegl Lek.* 2005;62(10):1176-9.

Krebs K. The spiritual aspect of caring—an integral part of health and healing. *Nurs Adm Q.* 2001 Spring;25(3):55-60.

Kreig M. *Black Market Medicine*. New York: Bantam, 1968.

Kübler-Ross E. *On Life After Death*. Berkeley, CA: Celestial Arts, 1991.

Kuo FF, Kuo JJ. *Recent Advances in Acupuncture Research, Institute for Adnanced Research in Asian Science and Medicine*. Garden City, New York. 1979.

Kwang Y, Cha , Daniel P, Wirth J, Lobo R. Does Prayer Influence the Success of *in Vitro*. Fertilization–Embryo Transfer? Report of a Masked, Randomized Trial. *J Reproductive Med.* 2001;46(9).

Lad V. *Ayurveda: The Science of Self-Healing*. Twin Lakes, WI: Lotus Press.

Lafrenière, G. The material Universe is made purely out of Aether. *Matter is made of Waves.* 2002. http://www.glafreniere.com/matter.htm. Acc. 2007 June.

Lakin-Thomas PL. Transcriptional feedback oscillators: maybe, maybe not. *J Biol Rhythms.* 2006 Apr;21(2):83-92.

Langhinrichsen-Rohling J, Palarea RE, Cohen J, Rohling ML. Breaking up is hard to do: unwanted pursuit behaviors following the dissolution of a romantic relationship. *Violence Vict.* 2000 Spring;15(1):73-90.

Latour E. Functional electrostimulation and its using in neurorehabilitation. *Ortop Traumatol Rehabil.* 2006 Dec 29;8(6):593-601.

Lazarou J, Pomeranz BH, Corey PN. Incidence of adverse drug reactions in hospitalized patients: a meta-analysis of prospective studies. *JAMA.* 1998 Apr.

Leape L. Lucian Leape on patient safety in U.S. hospitals. Interview by Peter I Buerhaus. *J Nurs Scholarsh.* 2004;36(4):366-70.

Leder D. Spooky actions at a distance: physics, psi, and distant healing. *J Altern Complement Med.* 2005 Oct;11(5):923-30.

Lewontin R. *The Genetic Basis of Evolutionary Change*. New York: Columbia Univ Press, 1974.

Li KH. Bioluminescence and stimulated coherent radiation. *Laser und Elektrooptik 3.* 1981:32-35.

Li N, Wang DL, Wang CW, Wu B. Discussion on randomized controlled trials about clinical researches of acupuncture and moxibustion medicine. *Zhongguo Zhen Jiu.* 2007 Jul;27(7):529-32.

Lipkind M. Can the vitalistic Entelechia principle be a working instrument ? (The theory of the biological field of Alexander G.Gurvich). In: Popp F, Li K, Gu Q (eds.). *Recent Advances in Biophoton Research*. Singapore: World Sci Publ, 1992:469-494.

Lipkind M. Registration of spontaneous photon emission from virus-infected cell cultures: development of experimental system. *Indian J Exp Biol.* 2003 May;41(5):457-72.

Lloyd D and Murray D. Redox rhythmicity: clocks at the core of temporal coherence. *BioEssays.* 2007;29(5): 465-473.

Lovelock J. *Gaia: A New Look at Life on Earth*. Oxford: Oxford Press, 1979.

Lovely RH. Recent studies in the behavioral toxicology of ELF electric and magnetic fields. *Prog Clin Biol Res.* 1988;257:327-47.

Lu J, Cui Y, Shi R. *A Practical English-Chinese Library of Traditional Chinese Medicine: Chinese Acupuncture and Moxibustion*. Shanghai: Publishing House of the Shanghai College of Traditional Chinese Medicine, 1988.

Lucas A, Morley R, Cole T, Lister G, Leeson-Payne C. Breast milk and subsequent intelligence quotient in children born premature. Lancet. 1992;339:261-264.

Lucas WB (ed). *Regression Therapy: A Handbook for Professionals. Past-Life Therapy*. Crest Park, CA: Deep Forest Press, 1993.

Lynch M, Walsh B. *Genetics and Analysis of Quantitative Traits*. Sunderland, MA: Sinauer, 1998

Lythgoe JN. Visual pigments and environmental light. *Vision Res.* 1984;24(11):1539-50.

Maas J, Jayson, J. K.. & Kleiber, D. A. Effects of spectral differences in illumination on fatigue. *J Appl Psychol.* 1974;59:524-526.

Maccabee PJ, Amassian VE, Cracco RQ, Cracco JB, Eberle L, Rudell A. Stimulation of the human nervous system using the magnetic coil. *J Clin Neurophysiol.* 1991 Jan;8(1):38-55.

MacDougall D. The Soul: Hypothesis Concerning Soul Substance Together with Experimental Evidence of The Existence of Such Substance. *J Am Soc Psych Res.* 1907 May.

MacKay D. *Science, Chance, and Providence.* Oxford: Oxford Univ Press, 1978.

MacKay D. *The Open Mind and Other Essays.* Downer's Grove, IL: Inter-Varsity Press, 1988.

Maes HH, Silberg JL, Neale MC, Eaves LJ. Genetic and cultural transmission of antisocial behavior: an extended twin parent model. *Twin Res Hum Genet.* 2007 Feb;10(1):136-50.

Magni P, Motta M, Martini L. Leptin: a possible link between food intake, energy expenditure, and reproductive function. *Regul Pept.* 2000 Aug 25;92(1-3):51-6.

Magnusson A, Stefansson JG. Prevalence of seasonal affective disorder in Iceland. *Arch Gen Psychiatry.* 1993 Dec;50(12):941-6.

Mahachoklertwattana P, Sudkronrayudh K, Direkwattanachai C, Choubtum L, Okascharoen C. Decreased cortisol response to insulin induced hypoglycaemia in asthmatics treated with inhaled fluticasone propionate. *Arch Dis Child.* 2004 Nov;89(11):1055-8.

Marks C. *Commissurotomy, Consciousness, and Unity of Mind.* Cambridge: MIT Press, 1981.

Marks L. *The Unity of the Senses: Interrelations among the Modalities.* New York: Academic Press, 1978.

Mastorakos G, Pavlatou M. Exercise as a stress model and the interplay between the hypothalamus-pituitary-adrenal and the hypothalamus-pituitary-thyroid axes. *Horm Metab Res.* 2005 Sep;37(9):577-84.

Matutinovic Z, Galic M. Relative magnetic hearing threshold. *Laryngol Rhinol Otol.* 1982 Jan;61(1):38-41.

Mayr E. *Toward a New Philosophy of Biology: Observations of an evolutionist.* Boston: Belknap Press, 1988.

Mayron L, Ott J, Nations R, Mayron E. Light, radiation and academic behaviour: Initial studies on the effects of full-spectrum lighting and radiation shielding on behaviour and academic performance of school children. *Acad Ther.* 1974;10, 33-47.

McConnel JV, Cornwell PR, Clay M. An apparatus for conditioning Planaria. *Am J Psychol.* 1960 Dec;73:618-22.

McCulloch M, Jezierski T, Broffman M, Hubbard A, Turner K, Janecki T. Diagnostic accuracy of canine scent detection in early- and late-stage lung and breast cancers. *Integr Cancer Ther.* 2006 Mar;5(1):30-9.

McTaggart L. *The Field.* New York: Quill, 2003.

Mead GRS. *Thrice-Greatest Hermes: Studies in Hellenistic Theosophy and Gnosis.* London: The Theosophical Publishing Society, 1906.

Medieval Sourcebook: Fifth Ecumenical Council. Constantinople II, 553

Meinecke FW. Sequelae and rehabilitation of spinal cord injuries. *Curr Opin Neurol Neurosurg.* 1991 Oct;4(5):714-9.

Melzack R, Coderre TJ, Katz J, Vaccarino AL. Central neuroplasticity and pathological pain. *Ann N Y Acad Sci.* 2001 Mar;933:157-74.

Melzack R, Wall PD. Pain mechanisms: a new theory. *Science.* 1965 Nov 19;150(699):971-9.

Melzack R. Evolution of the neuromatrix theory of pain. The prithvi raj lecture: presented at the third world congress of world institute of pain, barcelona 2004. *Pain Pract.* 2005 Jun;5(2):85-94.

Melzack R. Pain—an overview. *Acta Anaesthesiol Scand.* 1999 Oct;43(9):880-4.

Melzack R. Pain: past, present and future. *Can J Exp Psychol.* 1993 Dec;47(4):615-29.

Miller GT. *Living in the Environment.* Belmont, CA: Wadsworth, 1996.

Miller JD, Morin LP, Schwartz WJ, Moore RY. New insights into the mammalian circadian clock. *Sleep.* 1996 Oct;19(8):641-67.

Miller K. Cholesterol and In-Hospital Mortality in Elderly Patients. Am Family Phys. 2004 May.

Mills A. A replication study: Three cases of children in northern India who are said to remember a previous life," *J. Sci. Explor.* 1989;3(2):133-184.

Mills A. Moslem cases of the reincarnation type in northern India: A test of the hypothesis of imposed identification, Part I: Analysis of 26 cases. *J. Sci. Exploration.* 1990;4(2):171-188.

Mindell E, Hopkins V. *Prescription Alternatives.* New Canaan CT: Keats, 1998.

Mineev VN, Bulatova NI, Fedoseev GB. Erythrocyte insulin-reactive system and carbohydrate metabolism in bronchial asthma. *Ter Arkh.* 2002;74(3):14-7.

Mishkin M, Appenzeller T. The Anatomy of Memory. *Sci. Am.* 1987 June.

Mishkin M. Memory in monkeys severely impaired by combined but not by separate removal of amygdala and hippocampus. *Nature.* 1978;273: 297-298.

Mitchell JL. *Out-of-Body Experiences: A Handbook.* New York: Ballantine Books, 1981.

Miu AC, Benga O. Aluminum and Alzheimer's disease: a new look. *J Alzheimers Dis.* 2006 Nov;10(2-3):179-201.

Modern Biology. Austin: Harcourt Brace, 1993.

Monod J. *Chance and Necessity.* New York: Vintage, 1972.

Monroe R. *Far Journeys.* Garden City, NY: Doubleday & Co., 1985.

Monroe R. *Journeys Out of the Body.* Garden City, NY: Anchor Press, 1977.

Montanes P, Goldblum MC, Boller F. The naming impairment of living and nonliving items in Alzheimer's disease. *J Int Neuropsychol Soc.* 1995 Jan;1(1):39-48.

Moody R. *Coming Back: A Psychiatrist Explores Past-Life Journeys.* New York: Bantam Books, 1991.

Moody R. *Life After Life.* New York: Bantam, 1975.

Moody, R. *Reflections on Life After Life: More Important Discoveries In The Ongoing Investigation Of Survival Of Life After Bodily Death.* New York: Bantam, 1977.

Moore RY. Neural control of the pineal gland. *Behav Brain Res.* 1996;73(1-2):125-30.

Moore RY. Organization and function of a central nervous system circadian oscillator: the suprachiasmatic hypothalamic nucleus. *Fed Proc.* 1983 Aug;42(11):2783-9.

Morick H. *Introduction to the Philosophy of Mind: Readings from Descartes to Strawson.* Glenview, Ill: Scott Foresman, 1970.

Morse M. *Closer to the Light.* New York: Ivy Books, 1990.

Morton C. *Velocity Alters Electric Field.* www.amasci.com/ freenrg/ morton1.html. Accessed 2007 July.

Morton G. Hypothalamic Leptin Regulation of Energy Homeostasis and Glucose Metabolism. *J Physiol.* 2007 Jun 21.

Motoyama H. Acupuncture Meridians. *Science & Medicine.* 1999 July/August.

Motoyama H. Before Polarization Current and the Acupuncture Meridians. *Journal of Holistic Medicine.* 1986;8(1&2).

Motoyama H. Deficient/ Excessive Patterns Found in Meridian Functioning in Cases of Liver Disease. *Subtle Energy & Energy Medicine.* 2000; 11(2).

Motoyama H. Energetic Medicine: new science of healing: An interview with A. Jackson. www.shareintl.org/archives/health-healing/hh_adjenergetic.html. Acc. 2007 Oct.

Motoyama H. Smith, W. Harada T. Pre-Polarization Resistance of the Skin as Determined by the Single Square Voltage Pulse. *Psychophysiology.* 1984;21(5).

Muhlack S, Lemmer W, Klotz P, Muller T, Lehmann E, Klieser E. Anxiolytic effect of rescue remedy for psychiatric patients: a double-blind, placebo-controlled, randomized trial. *J Clin Psychopharmacol.* 2006 Oct;26(5):541-2.

Mumby DG, Wood ER, Pinel J. Object-recognition memory is only mildly impaired in rats with lesions of the hippocampus and amygdala. *Psychobio.* 1992;20: 18-27.

Murchie G. *The Seven Mysteries of Life.* Boston: Houghton Mifflin Company, 1978.

Musaev AV, Nasrullaeva SN, Zeinalov RG. Effects of solar activity on some demographic indices and morbidity in Azerbaijan with reference to A. L. Chizhevsky's theory. *Vopr Kurortol Fizioter Lech Fiz Kult.* 2007 May-Jun;(3):38-42.

Muzzarelli L, Force M, Sebold M. Aromatherapy and reducing preprocedural anxiety: A controlled prospective study. *Gastroenterol Nurs.* 2006 Nov-Dec;29(6):466-71.

Myss C. *Anatomy of the Spirit.* New York: Harmony, 1996.

Nadkarni AK, Nadkarni KM. *Indian Materia Medica*. (Vols 1 and 2). Bombay, India: Popular Pradashan, 1908, 1976.

Nakamura K, Urayama K, Hoshino Y. Lumbar cerebrospinal fluid pulse wave rising from pulsations of both the spinal cord and the brain in humans. *Spinal Cord*. 1997 Nov;35(11):735-9.

Nakatani K, Yau KW. Calcium and light adaptation in retinal rods and cones. *Nature*. 1988 Jul 7;334(6177):69-71.

Natarajan E, Grissom C. The Origin of Magnetic Field Dependent Recombination in Alkylcobalamin Radical Pairs. *Photochem Photobiol*. 1996;64: 286-295.

Navarro Silvera SA, Rohan TE. Trace elements and cancer risk: a review of the epidemiologic evidence. *Cancer Causes Control*. 2007 Feb;18(1):7-27.

Nestel PJ. Adulthood - prevention: Cardiovascular disease. *Med J Aust*. 2002 Jun 3;176(11 Suppl):S118-9.

Nestor PJ, Graham KS, Bozeat S, Simons JS, Hodges JR. Memory consolidation and the hippocampus: further evidence from studies of autobiographical memory in semantic dementia and frontal variant frontotemporal dementia. *Neuropsychologia*. 2002;40(6):633-54.

Netheron M. *Past Lives Therapy*. New York: Morrow, 1978.Wambach H. *Reliving Past Lives*. New York: Bantam, 1978.Fiore E. *You Have Been Here Before*. New York: Ballantine, 1978.

Newmark T, Schulick P. *Beyond Aspirin*. Prescott, AZ: Holm, 2000.

Newton M. *Destiny of Souls: New Case Studies of Life between Lives*. St. Paul: Llewellyn Publications, 2000.

Newton M. *Journey of Souls: Case Studies of Life between Lives*. St. Paul: Llewellyn Publications, 1994.

Newton PE. The Effect of Sound on Plant Grwoth. *JAES*. 1971 Mar;19(3): 202-205.

Nicholson A, Rose R, Bobak M. Association between attendance at religious services and self-reported health in 22 European countries. *Soc Sci Med*. 2009 Aug;69(4):519-28.

Niggli H. Temperature dependence of ultraweak photon emission in fibroblastic differentiation after irradiation with artificial sunlight. *Indian J Exp Biol*. 2003 May;41:419-423.

North J. *The Fontana History of Astronomy and Cosmology*. London: Fontana Press, 1994.

O'Dwyer JJ. *College Physics*. Pacific Grove, CA: Brooks/Cole, 1990.

O'Brien SJ, Shannon JE, Gail MH. A molecular approach to the identification and individualization of human and animal cells in culture: isozyme and allozyme genetic signatures. *In Vitro*. 1980 Feb;16(2):119-35.

O'Connor J., Bensky D. (ed). *Shanghai College of Traditional Chinese Medicine: Acupuncture: A Comprehensive Text*. Seattle: Eastland Press, 1981.

Onder G, Landi F, Volpato S, Fellin R, Carbonin P, Gambassi G, Bernabei R. Serum cholesterol levels and in-hospital mortality in the elderly. *Am J Med*. 2003 Sept;115:265-71

One Hundred Million Americans See Medical Mistakes Directly Touching Them as Patients, Friends, Relatives. *National Patient Safety Foundation. Press Release*. 1997 Oct 9. http://npsf.org/pr/pressrel/ finalsur.htm. Acc. 2007 Mar.

Oosterga M, ten Vaarwerk IA, DeJongste MJ, Staal MJ. Spinal cord stimulation in refractory angina pectoris — clinical results and mechanisms. *Z Kardiol*. 1997;86 Suppl 1:107-13.

Ostrander S, Schroeder L, Ostrander N. *Super-Learning*. New York: Delta, 1979.

Otani S. Memory trace in prefrontal cortex: theory for the cognitive switch. *Biol Rev Camb Philos Soc*. 2002 Nov;77(4):563-77.

Ott J. Color and Light: Their Effects on Plants, Animals, and People (Series of seven articles in seven issues). *Internl J Biosoc Res*. 1985-1991.

Ott J. *Health and Light: The Effects of Natural and Artificial Light on Man and Other Living Things*. Self published, 1973,

Park AE, Fernandez JJ, Schmedders K, Cohen MS. The Fibonacci sequence: relationship to the human hand. *J Hand Surg*. 2003 Jan;28(1):157-60.

Pasricha S. Cases of the reincarnation type in northern India with birthmarks and birth defects. *J. Sci. Exploration*. 1998;12(2) 259-293.

Pasricha S. *Claims of reincarnation: An Empirical Study of Cases in India*. New Delhi: Harman, 1990.

Penn RD, Hagins WA. Kinetics of the photocurrent of retinal rods. *Biophys J.* 1972 Aug;12(8):1073-94.

Penn RD, Hagins WA. Signal transmission along retinal rods and the origin of the electroretinographic a-wave. *Nature.* 1969 Jul 12;223(5202):201-4.

Penson RT, Kyriakou H, Zuckerman D, Chabner BA, Lynch TJ Jr. Teams: communication in multidisciplinary care. *Oncologist.* 2006 May;11(5):520-6.

Perry J. *A Dialogue on Personal Identity and Immortality.* Indianapolis, IN: Hackett, 1978.

Perry J. *Personal Identity.* Berkeley: University of California Press, 1975.

Persinger M.A. Psi phenomena and temporal lobe activity: The geomagnetic factor. In L.A. Henkel & R.E. Berger (Eds.), *Research in parapsychology.* (121- 156). Metuchen, NJ: Scarecrow Press, 1989.

Persinger M.A., Krippner S. Dream ESP experiments and geomagnetic activity. *Journal of the American Society of Psychical Research.* 1989;83:101- 106.

Persson R, Orbaek P, Kecklund G, Akerstedt T. Impact of an 84-hour workweek on biomarkers for stress, metabolic processes and diurnal rhythm. *Scand J Work Environ Health.* 2006 Oct;32(5):349-58.

Pert C. *Molecules of Emotion.* New York: Scribner, 1997.

Pew Foundation. Are We Happy Yet? *Pew Center Publications.* February 13, 2006

Physicians' Desk Reference. Montvale, NJ: Thomson, 2003.

Piolino P, Desgranges B, Belliard S, Matuszewski V, Lalevee C, De la Sayette V, Eustache F. Autobiographical memory and autonoetic consciousness: triple dissociation in neurodegenerative diseases. *Brain.* 2003 Oct;126(Pt 10):2203-19.

Pitt-Rivers R, Trotter WR. *The Thyroid Gland.* London: Butterworth Publisher, 1954.

Plotkin H. *Darwin Machines and the Nature of Knowledge: Concerning adaptations, instinct and the evolution of intelligence.* New York: Penguin, 1994.

Polkinghorne J. *Science and Providence.* Boston: Shambhala Publications, 1989.

Popp F Chang J. Mechanism of interaction between electromagnetic fields and living organisms. *Science in China.* 2000 Series C;43(5):507-518.

Popp F, Chang J, Herzog A, Yan Z, Yan Y. Evidence of non-classical (squeezed) light in biological systems. *Physics Lett.* 2002;293:98-102.

Popp F, Yan Y. Delayed luminescence of biological systems in terms of coherent states. *Phys.Lett.* 2000;293:91-97.

Popp F. Molecular Aspects of Carcinogenesis. In Deutsch E, Moser K, Rainer H, Stacher A (eds.). *Molecular Base of Malignancy.* Stuttgart: G.Thieme, 1976:47-55.

Popp F. Properties of biophotons and their theoretical implications. *Indian J Exper Biology.* 2003 May;41:391-402.

Popper KR, Eccles, JC. *The Self and Its Brain.* London: Routledge, 1983.

Prescott J. Alienation of Affection. *Psych Today.* 1979 Dec.

Prescott J. The Origins of Human Love and Violence. *Pre- and Perinatal Psych J.* 1996;10(3):143-188.

Pribram K. *Brain and perception: holonomy and structure in figural processing.* Hillsdale, N. J.: Lawrence Erlbaum Assoc., 1991.

Protheroe WM, Captiotti ER, Newsom GH. *Exploring the Universe.* Columbus, OH: Merrill, 1989,

Puthoff H, Targ R, May E. Experimental Psi Research: Implication for Physics. AAAS Proceedings of the 1979 Symposium on the Role of Consciousness in the Physical World. 1981.

Puthoff H, Targ R. A Perceptual Channel for Information Transfer Over Kilometer distances: Historical Perspective and Recent Research. Proc. *IEEE.* 1976;64(3):329-254.

Radin D. *The Conscious Universe.* San Francisco: HarperEdge, 1997.

Rapley G. Keeping mothers and babies together—breastfeeding and bonding. *RCM Midwives.* 2002 Oct;5(10):332-4.

Rappoport J. Both sides of the pharmaceutical death coin. *Townsend Letter for Doctors and Patients.* 2006 Oct.

Rawlings M. *Beyond Death's Door.* New York: Bantam, 1979.

Reger D, Goode S, Mercer E. *Chemistry: Principles & Practice*. Fort Worth, TX: Harcourt Brace, 1993.

Retallack D. *The Sound of Music and Plants*. Marina Del Rey, CA: Devorss, 1973.

Richards R. *Darwin and the Emergence of Evolutionary Theories of Mind and Behavior*. Chicago: Univ Chicago Press, 1987.

Rieder M. *Mission to Millboro*. Nevada City, CA: Blue Dolphin, 1995.

Rieder M. *Return to Millboro: The Reincarnation Drama Continues*. Nevada City, CA: Blue Dolphin, 1995.

Rietbrock N, Hamel M, Hempel B, Mitrovic V, Schmidt T, Wolf GK. Actions of standardized extracts of Crataegus berries on exercise tolerance and quality of life in patients with congestive heart failure. *Arzneimittelforschung*. 2001 Oct;51(10):793-8.

Rindos D. *The Origins of Agriculture: An evolutionary perspective*. Burlington, MA: Academic Press, 1984.

Ring K. *Life at Death: A Scientific Investigation of the Near-Death Experience*. New York: Quill, 1982.

Roach M. *Stiff: The Curious Lives of Human Cadavers*. New York: W.W. Norton, 2003.

Rodermel SR, Smith-Sonneborn J. Age-correlated changes in expression of micronuclear damage and repair in Paramecium tetraurelia. *Genetics*. 1977 Oct;87(2):259-74.

Rosenlund M, Picciotto S, Forastiere F, Stafoggia M, Perucci CA. Traffic-related air pollution in relation to incidence and prognosis of coronary heart disease. *Epidemiology*. 2008 Jan;19(1):121-8.

Routasalo P, Isola A. The right to touch and be touched. *Nurs Ethics*. 1996 Jun;3(2):165-76.

Roy M, Kirschbaum C, Steptoe A. Intraindividual variation in recent stress exposure as a moderator of cortisol and testosterone levels. *Ann Behav Med*. 2003 Dec;26(3):194-200.

Rubin E and Farber J. *Pathology 3rd Edition*. Lippincott-Raven, Philadelphia, PA, 1999.

Russ MJ, Clark WC, Cross LW, Kemperman I, Kakuma T, Harrison K. Pain and self-injury in borderline patients: sensory decision theory, coping strategies, and locus of control. *Psychiatry Res*. 1996 Jun 26;63(1):57-65.

Russek LG, Schwartz GE. Narrative descriptions of parental love and caring predict health status in midlife: a 35-year follow-up of the Harvard Mastery of Stress Study. *Altern Ther Health Med*. 1996 Nov;2(6):55-62.

Russell IJ. Advances in fibromyalgia: possible role for central neurochemicals. *Am J Med Sci*. 1998;315:377-84.

Sabom M. *Light and Death: One Doctor's Fascinating Account of Near Death Experiences*. Grand Rapids, MI: Zondervan Publishing, 1998.

Sabom M. *Recollections of Death: A Medical Investigation*. New York: Harper and Row, 1982.

Sacks O. *The Man Who Mistook his Wife for a Hat and Other Clinical Tales*. New York: Simon & Schuster, 1998.

Sahlin C, Pettersson FE, Nilsson LN, Lannfelt L, Johansson AS. Docosahexaenoic acid stimulates non-amyloidogenic APP processing resulting in reduced Abeta levels in cellular models of Alzheimer's disease. *Eur J Neurosci*. 2007 Aug;26(4):882-9.

Sanders R. Slow brain waves play key role in coordinating complex activity. *UC Berkeley News*. 2006 Sep 14.

Schanberg SM, Field TM. Sensory deprivation stress and supplemental stimulation in the rat pup and preterm human neonate. *Child Dev*. 1987 Dec;58(6):1431-47.

Schlebusch KP, Maric-Oehler W, Popp FA. Biophotonics in the infrared spectral range reveal acupuncture meridian structure of the body. *J Altern Complement Med*. 2005 Feb;11(1):171-3.

Schmidt H, Quantum processes predicted? *New Sci*. 1969 Oct 16.

Schmitt B, Frölich L. Creative therapy options for patients with dementia—a systematic review. *Fortschr Neurol Psychiatr*. 2007 Dec;75(12):699-707.

Scoville WB, Milner B. Loss of recent memory after bilateral hippocampal lesions. *J Neurol Neurosurg Psychiatry*. 1957;20:11-21.

Semenza C. Retrieval pathways for common and proper names. *Cortex*. 2006 Aug;42(6):884-91.

Senekowitsch F, Endler PC, Pongratz W, Smith CW. Hormone effects by CD record /replay. *FASEB J.* 1995:A12025.

Senior F. Fallout. *New York Mag.* 2003 Fall.

Serra-Valls A. Electromagnetic Industrion and the Conservation of Momentum in the Spiral Paradox. *Cornell University Library.* http://arxiv.org/ftp/physics/papers/0012/0012009.pdf. Acc. 2007 Jul.

Serway R. *Physicis For Scientists & Engineers.* Philadelphia: Harcourt Brace, 1992.

Shaffer D. *Developmental Psychology: Theory, Research and Applications.* Monterey, CA: Brooks/Cole, 1985.

Sharp KC. *After the Light.* New York: William Morrow & Co., 1995.

Shen YF, Goddard G. The short-term effects of acupuncture on myofascial pain patients after clenching. *Pain Pract.* 2007 Sep;7(3):256-64.

Shevelev IA, Kostelianetz NB, Kamenkovich VM, Sharaev GA. EEG alpha-wave in the visual cortex: check of the hypothesis of the scanning process. *Int J Psychophysiol.* 1991 Aug;11(2):195-201.

Shupak NM, Prato FS, Thomas AW. Human exposure to a specific pulsed magnetic field: effects on thermal sensory and pain thresholds. *Neurosci Lett.* 2004 Jun 10;363(2):157-62.

Sicher F, Targ E, Moore D, Smith H. A Randomized Double-Blind Study of the Effect of Distant Healing in a Population With Advanced AIDS. Western Journal of Medicine. 1998;169 Dec::356-363.

Siegfried J. Electrostimulation and neurosurgical measures in cancer pain. *Recent Results Cancer Res.* 1988;108:28-32.

Simpson G. *The Major Features of Evolution.* New York: Columbia Univ Press, 1953.

Smith CW. Coherence in living biological systems. *Neural Network World.* 1994:4(3):379-388.

Smith MJ. "Effect of Magnetic Fields on Enzyme Reactivity" in Barnothy M.(ed.), *Biological Effects of Magnetic Fields.* New York: Plenum Press, 1969.

Smith MJ. *The Influence on Enzyme Growth By the 'Laying on of Hands: Dimenensions of Healing.* Los Altos, California: Academy of Parapsychology and Medicine, 1973.

Smith-Sonneborn J. Age-correlated effects of caffeine on non-irradiated and UV-irradiated Paramecium Aurelia. *J Gerontol.* 1974 May;29(3):256-60.

Smith-Sonneborn J. DNA repair and longevity assurance in Paramecium tetraurelia. *Science.* 1979 Mar 16;203(4385):1115-7.

Snyder K. Researchers Produce Firsts with Bursts of Light: Team generates most energetic terahertz pulses yet, observes useful optical phenomena. *Press Release: Brookhaven National Laboratory.* 2007 July 24.

Soler M, Chandra S, Ruiz D, Davidson E, Hendrickson D, Christou G. A third isolated oxidation state for the Mn12 family of singl molecule magnets. *ChemComm;* 2000; Nov 22.

Soul Has Weight, Physician Thinks. *The New York Times.* 1907 March 11:5.

Southgate, D. Nature and variability of human food consumption. *Philosophical Transactions of the Royal Society of London.* 1991; B(334): 281-288.

Speed Of Light May Not Be Constant, Physicist Suggests. *Science Daily.* 1999 Oct 6. www.sciencedaily.com/releases/1999/10/991005114024.htm. Acc. 2007 Jun.

Spence A. *Basic Human Anatomy.* Menlo Park, CA: Benjamin/Commings, 1986.

Spetner L. *Not By Chance! -Shattering The Modern Theory of Evolution.* New York: The Judaica Press, 1997.

Spillane M. Good Vibrations, A Sound 'Diet' for Plants. *The Growing Edge.* 1991 Spring.

Squire LR, Zola-Morgan S. The medial temporal lobe memory system. *Science.* 1991;253(5026):1380-1386.

Stanford, C. B. The hunting ecology of wild chimpanzees: Implications for the evolutionary ecology of Pliocene hominids. *American Anthropologist.* 1996;98: 96-113.

Steck B. Effects of optical radiation on man. *Light Resch Techn.* 1982;14:130-141.

Steiner R. *Agriculture.* Kimberton, PA: Bio-Dynamic Farming, 1924-1993.

Stevenson I, Samararatne G. Three new cases of the reincarnation type in Sri Lanka with written records made before verification. *J. Sci. Exploration.* 1988;2(2): 217-238.

Stevenson I. American children who claim to remember previous lives. *J. Nervous and Mental Disease*. 1983;171:742-748.

Stevenson I. *Cases of the Reincarnation Type*. Charlottesville, VA: Univ Virginia Press. Vol. 1: *Ten Cases in India*, 1975. Vol. 2: *Ten Cases in Sri Lanka*, 1977. Vol. 3: *Twelve Cases in Lebanon and Turkey*, 1980. Vol. 4: *Twelve Cases in Thailand and Burma*, 1983.

Stevenson I. *Children Who Remember Previous Lives: A Question of Reincarnation*. Charlottesville, VA: Univ Virginia Press, 1987.

Stevenson I. *European Cases of the Reincarnation Type*. Jefferson, NC: McFarland and Co., 2003.

Stevenson I. *Reincarnation and Biology: A Contribution to the Etiology of Birthmarks and Birth Defects*. (2 volumes). Westport, CN: Praeger Publishers, 1997.

Stevenson I. *Twenty Cases Suggestive of Reincarnation*. New York: American Society for Psychical Research, 1967.

Stevenson I. *Where Reincarnation and Biology Intersect*. Westport, CN: Praeger, 1997.

Stojanovic MP, Abdi S. Spinal cord stimulation. *Pain Physician*. 2002 Apr;5(2):156-66.

Stoupel EG, Frimer H, Appelman Z, Ben-Neriah Z, Dar H, Fejgin MD, Gershoni-Baruch R, Manor E, Barkai G, Shalev S, Gelman-Kohan Z, Reish O, Lev D, Davidov B, Goldman B, Shohat M. Chromosome aberration and environmental physical activity: Down syndrome and solar and cosmic ray activity, Israel, 1990-2000. *Int J Biometeorol*. 2005 Sep;50(1):1-5.

Strange BA, Dolan RJ. Anterior medial temporal lobe in human cognition: memory for fear and the unexpected. *Cognit Neuropsychiatry*. 2006 May;11(3):198-218.

Suppes P, Han B, Epelboim J, Lu ZL. Invariance of brain-wave representations of simple visual images and their names. *Proc Natl Acad Sci Psych-BS*. 1999;96(25):14658-14663.

Szyf M, McGowan P, Meaney MJ. The social environment and the epigenome. *Environ Mol Mutagen*. 2008 Jan;49(1):46-60.

Tapsell LC, Hemphill I, Cobiac L, Patch CS, Sullivan DR, Fenech M, Roodenrys S, Keogh JB, Clifton PM, Williams PG, Fazio VA, Inge KE. Health benefits of herbs and spices: the past, the present, the future. *Med J Aust*. 2006 Aug 21;185(4 Suppl):S4-24.

Taraban M, Leshina T, Anderson M, Grissom C. Magnetic Field Dependence and the Role of electron spin in Heme Enzymes: Horseradish Peroxidase. *J. Am. Chem. Soc*. 1997;119: 5768-5769.

Targ R, Katra J, Brown D, Wiegand W. Viewing the future: A pilot study with an error-detecting protocol. *J Sci Expl*. 9:3:367-380, 1995.

Targ R, Puthoff H. Information transfer under conditions of sensory shielding. *Nature*. 1975;251:602-607.

Taylor A. *Soul Traveler: A Guide to Out-of-Body Experiences and the Wonders Beyond*. New York: Penguin, 2000.

Thaut MH. The future of music in therapy and medicine. *Ann N Y Acad Sci*. 2005 Dec;1060:303-8.

The Timechart Company. *Timetables of Medicine*. New York: Black Dog & Leventhal, 2000.

Thie J. *Touch for Health*. Marina del Rey, CA: Devorss Publications, 1973-1994.

Thomas Y, Schiff M, Litime M, Belkadi L, Benveniste J. Direct transmission to cells of a molecular signal (phorbol myristate acetate, PMA) via an electronic device. *FASEB Jnl*. 1995;9: A227.

Thomas-Anterion C, Jacquin K, Laurent B. Differential mechanisms of impairment of remote memory in Alzheimer's and frontotemporal dementia. *Dement Geriatr Cogn Disord*. 2000 Mar-Apr;11(2):100-6.

Thompson D. *On Growth and Form*. Cambridge: Cambridge University Press, 1992.

Thorogood M, Mann J, Appleby P, McPherson K. Risk of death from cancer and ischaemic heart disease in meat and non-meat eaters. *BMJ*. 1994 June 25;308:1667-1670.

Threlkeld DS, ed. Central Nervous System Drugs, Analeptics, Caffeine. *Facts and Comparisons Drug Information*. St. Louis, MO: Facts and Comparisons. 1998 Feb: 230-d.

Threlkeld DS, ed. Gastrointestinal Drugs, Proton Pump Inhibitors. *Facts and Comparisons Drug Information*. St. Louis, MO: Facts and Comparisons. 1998 Apr: 305r.

Timofeev I, Steriade M. Low-frequency rhythms in the thalamus of intact-cortex and decorticated cats. *J Neurophysiol*. 1996 Dec;76(6):4152-68.

Ting W, Schultz K, Cac NN, Peterson M, Walling HW. Tanning bed exposure increases the risk of malignant melanoma. Int J Dermatol. 2007 Dec;46(12):1253-7.

Tompkins, P, Bird C. *The Secret Life of Plants*. New York: Harper & Row, 1973.

Toomer G. "Ptolemy". *The Dictionary of Scientific Biography*. New York: Gale Cengage, 1970.

Trivedi B. Magnetic Map" Found to Guide Animal Migration. *Natl Geogr Today*. 2001 Oct 12.

Tsong T. Deciphering the language of cells. *Trends in Biochem Sci*. 1989;14: 89-92.

Tsuei JJ, Lam Jr. F, Zhao Z. Studies in Bioenergetic Correlations-Bioenergetic Regulatory Measurement Instruments and Devices. *Am J Acupunct*. 1988;16:345-9.

Tucker J. *Life Before Life: A Scientific Investigation of Children's Memories of Previous Lives*. New York: St. Martin's Press, 2005.

Unger RH. Leptin physiology: a second look. *Regul Pept*. 2000 Aug 25;92(1-3):87-95.

Van Cauter E, Leproult R, Plat L. Age-related changes in slow wave sleep and REM sleep and relationship with growth hormone and cortisol levels in healthy men. *JAMA*. 2000 Aug 16;284(7):861-8.

Van Wijk R, Wiegant FAC. *Cultured mammalian cells in homeopathy research: the similia principle in self-recovery*. Utrecht: University Utrecht Publ, 1994.

Vargha-Khadem F, Polkey CE. A review of cognitive outcome after hemidecortication in humans. *Adv Exp Med Biol*. 1992;325:137-51.

Vierling-Claassen D, Siekmeier P, Stufflebeam S, Kopell N. Modeling GABA alterations in schizophrenia: a link between impaired inhibition and altered gamma and beta range auditory entrainment. *J Neurophysiol*. 2008 May;99(5):2656-71.

Vigny P, Duquesne M. *On the fluorescence properties of nucleotides and polynucleotides at room temperature*. In: Birks J (ed.). Excited states of biological molecules. London-NY: J Wiley, 1976:167-177.

Voll R. The phenomenon of medicine testing in elecroacupuncture according to Voll. *Am J Acupunct*. 1980;8:97-104.

Vyasadeva S. *Srimad Bhagavatam*. Approx rec 4000 B.C.E.

Wachiuli M, Koyama M, Utsuyama M, Bittman BB, Kitagawa M, Hirokawa K. Recreational music-making modulates natural killer cell activity, cytokines, and mood states in corporate employees. *Med Sci Monit*. 2007 Feb;13(2):CR57-70.

Wade N. From Ants to Ethics: A Biologist Dreams of Unity of Knowledge. Scientist at Work, Edward O. Wilson. *New York Times*. 1998 May 12.

Walker M. *The Power of Color*. Gujarat, India: Jain Publ., 2002.

Walsh DM, Selkoe DJ. A beta oligomers - a decade of discovery. *J Neurochem*. 2007 Jun;101(5):1172-84.

Watson L. *Beyond Supernature*. New York: Bantam, 1987.

Wayne R. *Chemistry of the Atmospheres*. Oxford Press, 1991.

Weaver J, Astumian R. The response of living cells to very weak electric fields: the thermal noise limit. *Science*. 1990;247: 459-462.

Wee K, Rogers T, Altan BS, Hackney SA, Hamm C. Engineering and medical applications of diatoms. *J Nanosci Nanotechnol*. 2005 Jan;5(1):88-91.

Weinberger P, Measures M. The effect of two audible sound frequencies on the germination and growth of a spring and winter wheat. *Can. J. Bot*. 1968;46(9):1151-1158.

Weiss B. *Many Lives, Many Masters*. New York: Simon & Schuster, 1988.

Weller A, Weller L. Menstrual synchrony between mothers and daughters and between roommates. *Physiol Behav*. 1993 May;53(5):943-9.

Weller L, Weller A, Roizman S. Human menstrual synchrony in families and among close friends: examining the importance of mutual exposure. *J Comp Psychol*. 1999 Sep;113(3):261-8.

Welsh D, Yoo SH, Liu A, Takahashi J, Kay S. Bioluminescence Imaging of Individual Fibroblasts Reveals Persistent, Independently Phased Circadian Rhythms of Clock Gene Expression. *Current Biology*. 2004;14:2289-2295.

White J, Krippner S (eds). *Future Science: Life Energies & the Physics of Paranormal Phenomena*. Garden City: Anchor, 1977.

White S. *The Unity of the Self*. Cambridge: MIT Press, 1991.

Whiten, A. and E. M. Widdowson (eds.). *Foraging Strategies and Natural Diet of Monkeys, Apes and Humans.* Oxford: Clarendon Press, 1991.

Whitfield KE, King G, Moller S, Edwards CL, Nelson T, Vandenbergh D. Concordance rates for smoking among African-American twins. *J Natl Med Assoc.* 2007 Mar;99(3):213-7.

Whittaker E. *History of the Theories of Aether and Electricity.* New York: Nelson LTD, 1953.

Whitton J. *Life Between Life.* New York: Warner, 1986.

Williams G. *Natural Selection: Domains, levels, and challenges.* Oxford: Oxford Univ Press, 1992.

Winchester AM. *Biology and its Relation to Mankind.* New York: Van Nostrand Reinhold, 1969.

Winter L, Dennis MP, Parker B. Preferences for life-prolonging medical treatments and deference to the will of god. *J Relig Health.* 2009 Dec;48(4):418-30.

Wixted JT. A Theory About Why We Forget What We Once Knew. *CurrDir Psychol Sci.* 2005;14(1):6-9.

Wolf, M. Beyond the Point Particle - *A Wave Structure for the Electron. Galilean Electrodynamics.* 1995 Oct;6(5): 83-91.

Woolger R. *Other Lives, Other Selves.* New York: Bantam, 1988.

Wyart C, Webster WW, Chen JH, Wilson SR, McClary A, Khan RM, Sobel N. Smelling a single component of male sweat alters levels of cortisol in women. *J Neurosci.* 2007 Feb 7;27(6):1261-5.

Yang HQ, Xie SS, Hu XL, Chen L, Li H. Appearance of human meridian-like structure and acupoints and its time correlation by infrared thermal imaging. *Am J Chin Med.* 2007;35(2):231-40.

Zhang C, Popp, F., Bischof, M.(eds.). *Electromagnetic standing waves as background of acupuncture system. Current Development in Biophysics - the Stage from an Ugly Duckling to a Beautiful Swan.* Hangzhou: Hangzhou University Press, 1996.

Zou Z, Li F, Buck L. Odor maps in the olfactory cortex. *Proc Natl Acad of Sci.* 2005;102(May 24):7724-7729.

Index

Lightning Source UK Ltd.
Milton Keynes UK
09 March 2011

168981UK00001B/44/P